What It Takes to Feel Good

THE NICKOLAUS TECHNIQUE

WHAT
IT TAKES
TO FEEL
GOOD

The Nickolaus

BENNO ISAACS and

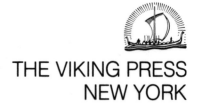

THE VIKING PRESS
NEW YORK

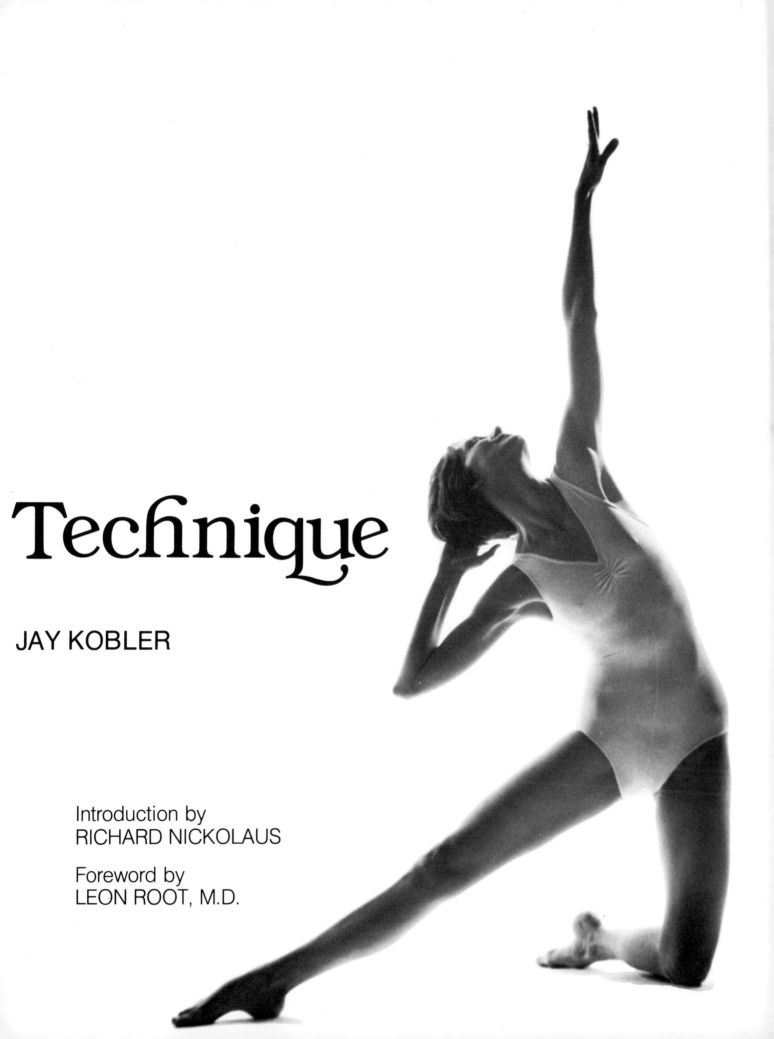

Technique

JAY KOBLER

Introduction by
RICHARD NICKOLAUS

Foreword by
LEON ROOT, M.D.

Copyright © Richard Nickolaus Ltd., 1978
All rights reserved
First published in 1978 by The Viking Press
625 Madison Avenue, New York, N.Y. 10022

Published simultaneously in Canada by
Penguin Books Canada Limited

Library of Congress Cataloging in Publication Data
Isaacs, Benno.
What it takes to feel good.

1. Exercise. I. Kobler, Jay, joint author.
II. Title.
RA781.I78   613.7'1   78-5349
ISBN 0-670-75824-8

Printed in the United States of America
Set in VIP Primer with Bookman Light
and Helvetica by Publishers Phototype, Inc.

Third printing October, 1978

Photographs on pages iii, 8, 20, 47, 50-53, 57-59, 66-81, 83,
94-97, 100-101, 106-109, 112-17, 120-21, 124-25, 129-31,
135, 138, and 145 by Bob Monckton. Photographs on pages 2,
26, and 40 by Kevin Higgins. Photograph on page 34 by Kenn
Duncan.

A short excerpt from this book appeared in *Woman's Day*.

THIS BOOK IS
DEDICATED TO
THE MILLIONS OF
PEOPLE WHO
CARE ABOUT
THEIR BODIES
AND MINDS.

FOREWORD

To the casual eye, the Nickolaus exercises in this book may look like a ballet dancer's plot to undermine your back. They are anything but.

They represent a good, sensible conditioning program. Done on a regular basis, they should, among other things, improve posture, help prevent fatigue, and restore muscle tone.

As an orthopedic surgeon who has had back pain, I am pleased to see that many of these exercises are aimed at giving that sensitive area of the body the help it needs to stay healthy.

The average American, softened by modern technology, which increasingly limits his or her physical activity, must think in terms of getting more exercise. It is important not only for the back, but for total physical and mental well-being.

Consequently, after a critical review of the Nickolaus Technique, I can recommend it as an intelligent approach to physical fitness. Of course you should consult your own physician before you embark on *any* course of physical exercise; but my suggestion is that you look into the Nickolaus Technique to see what it holds for you. It certainly can't hurt, and it is likely to help. You'll discover the only "plot" here is, with your cooperation, to make you feel good.

Leon Root, M.D.
New York Hospital for Special Surgery

ACKNOWLEDGMENTS

The authors wish to express their appreciation to the staff, instructors, and students of the Nickolaus Exercise Centers for their cooperation in the preparation of this book. Special thanks are due Richard Reiniger, president and owner of Richard Nickolaus, Ltd.; Margot Reiniger, who gave freely of her time and sensitive advice; and Paula Miksic, head receptionist for the Centers, whose help and patience made the authors' work much easier.

They are also deeply grateful to Viking editor Amanda Vaill, designer Barbara Knowles, and their agent, Roberta Kent, whose commitment to the project from the very beginning assured its success.

Finally, and particularly, they would like to thank Richard Nickolaus, whose hard work and breadth of vision in creating the Nickolaus Technique made writing this book a pleasure, and William Thompson, who contributed many valuable comments on the text of the book and the background of the Technique.

Richard Nickolaus wants to offer his own special thanks:

To the authors, for helping to validate the

Nickolaus Technique by relating it to scientific, medical, and psychological theory.

To Bill Thompson and Margot Reiniger, whose minds and bodies were indispensable in developing the Technique.

Above all to his wife, Harriett, without whose encouragement and support the first Nickolaus Exercise Center would have been impossible.

CONTENTS

What It Takes to Feel Good

THE NICKOLAUS TECHNIQUE

Introduction

by RICHARD NICKOLAUS

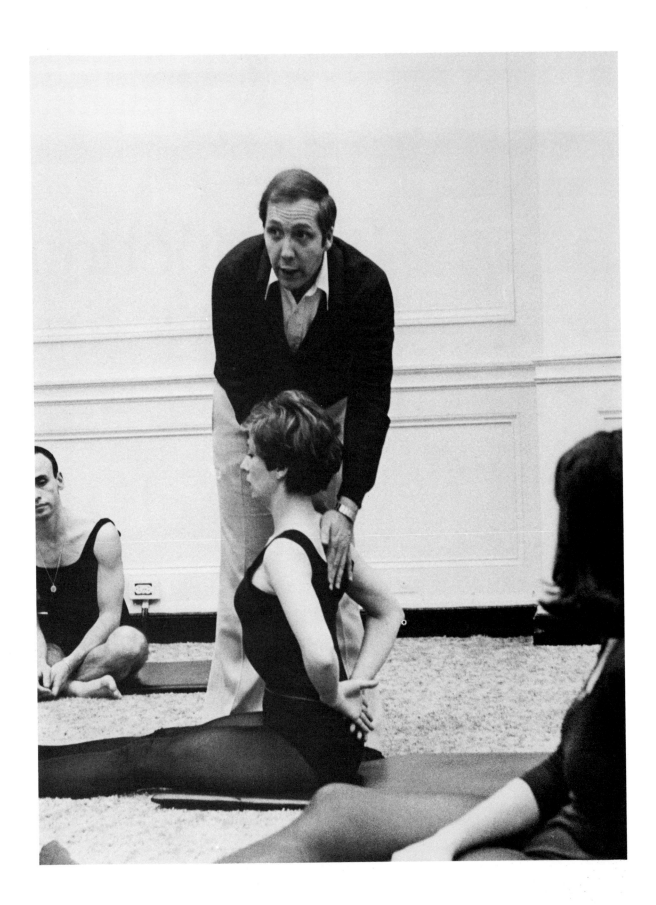

The Nickolaus Technique is a program of thirty sequenced exercises animated by the pulses of rhythm and breathing. It contains nearly half a lifetime of experience in the relationship of the human body to the total quality of human life. After an hour with the Nickolaus Technique, you will have exercised, without strain, as totally as if you had spent an hour at the ballet bar — with one crucial difference: The Technique improves body alignment by means of exercise done almost entirely on the floor, using your own body as the resistance rather than working against the forces of gravity.

This book tries to place the Nickolaus Technique within a framework of sound theory. I wish I could say the Technique evolved within that framework; the truth is, it was largely the result of practical day-to-day work with the body. To a great extent, it grew out of the problems and challenges I encountered as a choreographer. I could see that what I was doing worked; other people told me it worked; but it's only recently that I am beginning truly to grasp *why* it works.

From the outset, my own approach tended to be practical and intuitive. Among my first memories is a sense of pleasure in experiencing my body in motion. As I grew older, that feeling crystallized in the desire to dance; inevitably, I became a dancer.

After three years with the Cornish School of Allied Arts in Seattle, I came to New York City to study, and here the first thing I learned was that there were many different approaches to the study of ballet—many different methods of teaching—and that those differences were tremendously important in their impact on the student.

Most of the teachers I encountered didn't really seem to have a sound idea of how the body works. What they had to communicate was presented in an almost mystical way: Either you got it or you didn't—and if you got it, it was usually through endless repetition, rather than through any reasoned explanation of what was happening.

The dancer is studying an art technique, not a physical culture. Ballet exercises— *pliés*, *développées*, and so on—and performance are no more a preparation for being a dancer than running onto a tennis court and starting to hit a ball around is preparation for being a tennis player. Increasingly, I became aware of the need for a technique for getting the body together that would come *before* using the body in dance—or in any concentrated activity, for that matter.

When I'd been in New York about a year, I had dramatic proof of the need for such preparation. In class, I executed a movement incorrectly—and fractured my ankle. I was in a cast for nine months. The medical verdict: I would never dance again, nor even walk without a brace.

As part of my therapy, I was sent to Carola Trier, who taught a system of exercise using the Joseph Pilates apparatus. Even though I was overweight and sadly out of shape from those nine months of inactivity, three months with this wonderful teacher transformed me, put my body in the finest condi-

tion it had ever known. I regained the use of my ankle, and in addition I acquired a new understanding of my body and how to develop it. Hoping to master the exercise technique that had been so beneficial to me, I continued to work with Carola Trier and through her met the late Dr. Henry Jordan, head orthopedic surgeon at Lenox Hill Hospital in New York. With him I was able to observe firsthand the rehabilitation of patients suffering from all kinds of injury and illness, and I began to see that though it still wasn't possible for me to dance properly, there was nothing to prevent me from using my newfound knowledge as a dance teacher and choreographer. Working with Carola, I had met another dancer and choreographer named Bill Thompson, who—as it turned out—shared my frustration over the lack of system in dance training; we were both convinced that there must be a better, more precise way of teaching this precise and beautiful performing art.

With that conviction in mind, we created the American Choreographic Company; Bill was principal dancer, and one of our "discoveries" was Margot Travers (now Margot Reiniger), a young dancer who today is the prime example of the Nickolaus Technique in action, as you may gather from many of the illustrations accompanying the text of this book. Together we toured and lectured here and abroad, and worked with singers, actors, and musicians as well as dancers.

With this background, Bill and I opened the Montreal Dance Center; using springs and weights, I continued my experiments on the most effective way to train dancers. Gradually, we found we were employing more exercise movements and fewer dance movements in preparation for performance.

At this point, I should stress that we did not set out to become physical culturists. The Nickolaus Exercise Centers that eventually evolved from these early experiments were, in a sense, a spin-off from our efforts to be dancers and choreographers.

However, because so many dancers incur injuries, we began of necessity to work with orthopedic problems. Our work attracted some attention, and a woman with multiple sclerosis came to us with her doctor's permission to see if my exercises could improve her condition. Her muscles could not always obey the commands she gave them. For example, she could lift her damaged leg only once or twice off the ground before it stopped receiving signals. With exercise, she was able to achieve fifteen repetitions.

This seemed to indicate something crucial: If a group of muscles can't perform, the nervous system has the capacity to reroute signals. Although the damage can't be undone, it seems possible to compensate for damaged muscles with new thought and nerve patterns.

Later, I observed that the same principle could be successfully applied to scoliosis, a not uncommon back condition resulting from severe lateral curvature of the spine. Once scoliosis has occurred, it is not reversible; but the body can be trained to fight against the curvature and, in effect, provide its own brace.

My way to these findings was, again, practical and intuitive; our primary interest was still performance. Before long, we formed another ballet company and returned to the United States, where we were offered a short "artists' residence" at Duke University. Suddenly, it seemed everything I had observed and experienced for twelve years had come together; one evening in conversation with Bill Thompson, the entire basis of what would be the Nickolaus Technique emerged in about forty-five minutes. It still needed extensive testing.

At Duke, we mounted some new dance works and, most important, we had a chance to teach my exercises to a new audience of nondancers, including football players and other students. We soon opened the first "Nickolaus Center" in Durham, and there — with Jack Prost, a young doctor on the Duke faculty, on hand to answer our many questions about anatomy and physical capability — we began to test the Technique in practice, working with people who had various orthopedic problems, as well as with a child with severe scoliosis, a singer with a collapsed lung, and another woman with multiple sclerosis.

In every case, the exercises helped these people to overcome their problems. My practical curiosity was satisfied enough so that I felt ready to go ahead and start teaching full time.

So in 1972, the first professional center based on the Nickolaus Technique was opened in a church on Ninth Avenue in New York City. Now, six years later, the Technique is taught to over 3000 students in fourteen Exercise Centers — and the list is growing.

Perhaps one reason students come back time after time is that the Technique helps them to feel good. As one student, a model who originally came in with an injured knee, said to me: "Once I got into the routine of taking regular classes, I started feeling better all over, looking better, and feeling different about myself. Once you get the feeling you have some control over your body, you start feeling more confident. After all, how can you control a situation if you can't control your own body?"

Another student, a middle-aged insurance broker, put it another way: "Since I've gotten into the swing of the exercises, my back and neck don't bother me any more. Not only that, but I've been feeling so marvelously relaxed that I've got more energy — maybe it's because I'm not fighting the back pain constantly. I'll say this, too — once you get into the Nickolaus Technique, you don't want to stop because you feel so good."

And one convert spoke for many when she admitted: "After a time, doing the same exercises time and again can get boring. But making a regular thing of the exercises is addictive — it gets to be something you have to do and simply don't feel well not doing. So, when I do the exercises I'm bored, but when I don't do them there seems to be something missing. Maybe that's what life is all about. I simply don't know the answer."

The fact remains that exercise is still something most people just don't want to do. What makes the Nickolaus Technique so palatable is that it *is* a technique: You can feel the movements, the little improvements, each time you perform the exercises. You can feel the stress. Sometimes it will be tiring, even a little painful. But working so closely and intimately with your body can be enjoyable. And when you do the exercises regularly and properly, you should have absolutely no aches and pains or stiffness later on. In fact, it's virtually guaranteed that you'll feel better after your workout.

All this may seem a long-winded prologue to what is essentially a series of thirty exercises, but I think it is important for you to have some idea of how these exercises came to be developed. They are the result of observing what the body actually does, and what works to support the body and prepare it for its action in daily life.

For that reason, they really work. Each movement in the Technique is designed to exercise a specific part of the body — to tone and refine every muscle individually and all muscles together. Performed properly, in the correct sequence and supported by the system of deep breathing described in this book, the exercises can improve your body alignment, tone your muscles, strengthen problem areas like the back and the knees, increase flexibility, and even reduce physical and mental tension.

The connection between body and mind is probably the factor most frequently overlooked in exercise programs. Stimulating the body will also stimulate the brain, release tension in the muscles, activate glands, and coordinate the nervous system. The most common feeling expressed by students at the end of a session in a Nickolaus Exercise Center is one of exhilaration.

With a set discipline of only two hours a week, you can prepare yourself for a broad range of tasks — skiing, tennis, dancing, even childbirth — while becoming more in touch with your body, mind, instincts, and emotions.

Feeling Good

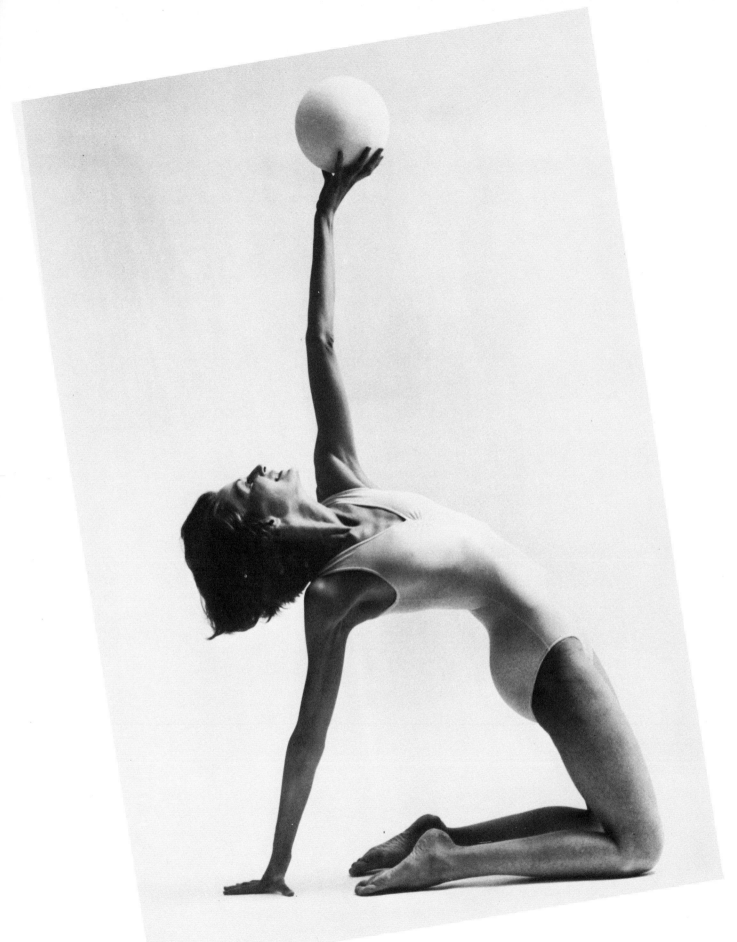

Television commercials have acquainted us only too thoroughly with the ills to which the flesh and mind of modern man are heir: back pain, headaches, tension, dizziness, lack of energy, anxiety, "the blahs."

If you suffer from any or all of those conditions, the chances are overwhelming that at least part of the problem can be attributed to lack of exercise.

Nineteen centuries ago, the Romans had a saying that expressed their attitude toward people's responsibility for their lives: "Man does not die, he kills himself." This sounds like a pretty negative approach to life until you consider its logical reverse: We can also choose *not* to kill ourselves.

Of course, making that choice presupposes an awareness that a choice exists and that there is some urgency about making it. Most people have a sort of vague idea that exercise is good for them and that they aren't getting enough of it, but it has only recently become apparent that few Americans are really aware how much better they could be feeling most of the time, and how important the condition of the body is in achieving that improvement. A recent Roper survey found that more than half the patients who have physical checkups in this country are warned about their body's condition by the doctors who examine them. In most cases, they are advised to develop a regular regimen of exercise — "or else."

For Americans at least, the problem begins early in life. A well-publicized study of physical strength and ability among young Americans, reported more than twenty years ago and based on fifteen years of research, showed that American children were in dramatically poor condition, as compared with their European counterparts. This benchmark study, undertaken by Dr. Hans Kraus and Dr. Sonja Weber in the posture clinic of New York's Columbia Presbyterian Medical Center, was based on physical fitness tests given to 4264 children in this country and 2870 in Austria, Italy, and Switzerland.

Despite the higher standard of living and greater access to exercise facilities in the United States, American youth lagged far behind Europeans in physical fitness: Of six tests for muscular strength and flexibility, nearly six in ten American children failed one or more, while less than one in ten of the European youngsters failed one or more.

And the President's Council of Physical Fitness and Sports believes that situation is no better today. People who *were* in good physical condition when they were young are letting themselves get out of shape. All through high school or college they are likely to participate in a regular exercise or athletic program, but once out, they stop abruptly. A common case is the person who sits behind a desk five days a week, then on the weekend participates in strenuous activity. That's the person you'll see in the doctor's office on Monday morning.

In a sense, exercise is natural. Animals do it; watch kittens stretching, tumbling, hurling themselves into endless mock battles. Even in confinement animals will race or pace round and round their cages, driven by the need to keep their bodies active.

Unfortunately, in the human animal that need often becomes numbed and blunted by a different sort of confinement, and exercise can come to feel quite "unnatural." We are, in a sense, prisoners of a daily life that offers no incentive and few means to develop and maintain good muscle tone or cardiovascular and respiratory fitness. Machines have just about made it unnecessary to walk long distances, climb stairs, or carry heavy objects, as well as to rely on physical activity for entertainment. One machine, the TV set, holds children spellbound and inactive for what one estimate puts at as long as fifty hours a week.

Our bodies are victims of progress. Generally speaking, today it is only the laborer or blue-collar worker who has to use his body on the job. Nearly everyone else, with the exception of the professional athlete or dancer, has no "need" to maintain his muscles.

Even the typical professional athlete or blue-collar worker does not exercise his body frequently or well enough to maintain the kind of muscle tone that can consistently support his activity without inviting injury to the body.

Modern men and women lead faster lives than their ancestors; ironically, their bodies are less well equipped to deal with that frenzied pace.

It is not going too far to say we have been "disconnected" from our bodies by the rapidity with which our working environment has evolved. Barely a century ago, fields were tilled by men and animals, and the furnaces of industry were stoked by muscle power. Today, the muscular, respiratory, and circulatory systems of the human body are still designed for, and still require, regular and vigorous use, but the typical job in a modern office or automated factory requires less physical energy than taking a hot shower does.

For machines and electrical conveniences, by removing the necessity for us to use our bodies, can also remove our *ability* to use them — or control them.

The American kitchen and home, too, are so full of gadgets and electrical motors that, despite a heavy schedule and frenzied activity, the housewife isn't apt to get much benefit out of her physical chores. In fact, if she hasn't prepared herself with a program of exercise that makes her conscious of how her body operates, the household tasks she performs every day may break her down rather than build her up.

As our work habits have changed, so have our eating habits: In the past twenty years we've begun to eat an increasing amount of prepared foods, including pre-concocted meals and synthetic imitations of the real thing, many with lists of artificial ingredients that would make a chemist's tongue curl.

This is not a book about diet, but the subject is almost unavoidable in any consideration of the body. The sad fact is that most Americans eat the wrong things, in the wrong quantity, at the wrong time — and, as a result, about seventy million people in the United States (according to one estimate) are overweight.

Poor eating habits severely compound the problems resulting from inadequate exercise. The excess weight caused by sedentary living and overeating can lead to heart trouble, arteriosclerosis, high blood pressure, and diabetes; and although it has been stated in some medical circles that exercise per se has no direct effect on the regulation of weight, it *does*.

Studies by the eminent nutritionist Dr. Jean Mayer show that when daily physical activity drops to a certain low level — below the equivalent of a two-mile daily walk, approximately — the brain's appetite regulators go haywire and tell the body it's hungry when it's not. In other words, the less you exercise, the more you want to eat.

So far we've considered exercise from the somewhat negative standpoint of why we don't get enough of it. More important and, for most people, more convincing are the positive benefits of exercise they realize from the Nickolaus Technique. Exercise doesn't stop with its immediate impact on the body — it affects our minds, emotions, and effectiveness. When you are fit, your fitness is transformed into energy, allowing you to handle problems and tackle projects head-on. If you are fit, you get more done in less time. You are more positive, you cope better under stress, and you are sick less often. If you follow a regular, individual exercise program, it can serve as an energizing "rest break" in the work day. The more sedentary and cerebral your job is, the more of those rest breaks you need.

The Nickolaus Technique follows directly on the latest experiments and theories of health experts. There is increasing evidence that exercise produces physiological changes that have a direct bearing on emotional factors. In fact, exercise may even cause chemical changes in the brain that actually alter thinking. Basically, brain function depends on nourishment. The blood supplies the necessary brain food — oxygen — and removes waste products. Since exercise increases the blood flow, more nutrients reach the brain cells.

Oxygen is the most important element in the brain's function. Insufficient oxygen results in a decline of intellect and reasoning power, a condition that can be improved only by adding oxygen — as a group of clinical psychologists at the Veterans Administration Hospital in Buffalo, New York, discovered when they administered large amounts of pure oxygen to senile patients and noted an increase in the patients' mental alertness.

Vigorous exercise — especially when coupled, as in the Nickolaus Technique, with attention to correct breathing—increases lung capacity eight to ten times. That means more oxygen enters the lungs. The actual capacity of the blood to carry that essential fuel is also increased, due to a greater amount of hemoglobin in the bloodstream. So the brain gets the oxygen it needs, and then some.

The effect of exercise on the mind goes beyond the simple link between oxygen and brain condition, though. If you do it regularly, exercise gives you a degree of protection by conditioning your body's stress mechanism. When you are fit, you build up a better reserve of hormonelike chemicals, such as adrenaline, which help the body overcome prolonged tension. You also will have a lower level of serum triglycerides—which have been linked in several studies with cholesterol as a significant factor in heart trouble—and your blood pressure will be more likely to stay within manageable limits. And it's widely accepted by psychologists that exercise releases nervous tension and anxiety by providing an outlet for pent-up aggression and hostility.

None of that should be difficult to accept in theory, though it's not so easy to translate into what happens in our lives from day to day. But studies in the Soviet Union have shown that, other things being equal, workers who participated in exercise drills had a higher working capacity. The rate of their output was two to five percent, and sometimes ten to fifteen percent, higher than that of nonathletes. What's more, people who participated in sports consulted doctors four times less often than those who did not participate, and workers who exercised regularly fell ill three to four times less frequently than those of the same age who didn't. For middle-aged and elderly people, the difference was five to eight times less often.

Today, increasing numbers of men and women realize that, besides trimming muscles and streamlining one's body, a personal physical fitness program is the best way of encouraging good health, physical and mental. If you're reading this book, you're probably one of those people. And that's what the Nickolaus Technique is all about.

A
Beautiful
Well-Balanced
Machine

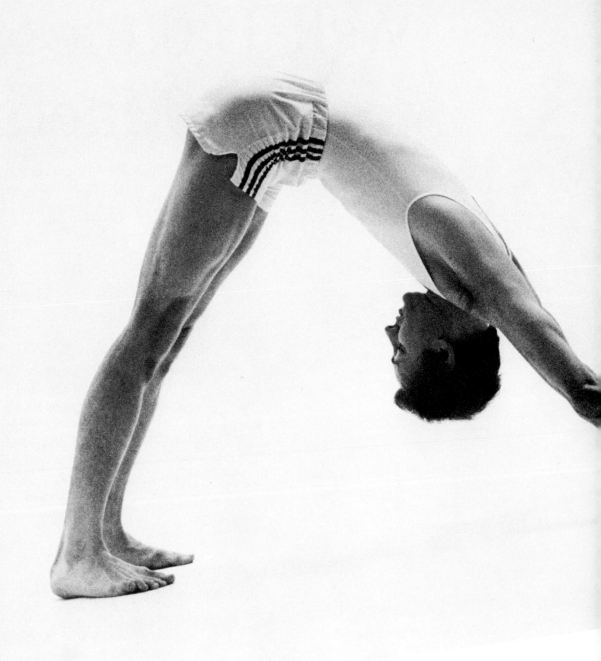

When you think of exercise, do you think of physical-training calisthenics: swinging from parallel bars, twisting the body into pretzel shapes? Actually, anything that requires movement is exercise. Walking, sitting, and standing, we exercise whether we know it or not.

There may, however, be immense differences from one person to another in the quality and effect of that exercise; for when a muscle works, many more things happen than the simple movement.

First, like any machine or organism, the muscle demands energy, and it produces waste as a by-product of its function. And the body itself supplies the energy in the form of glucose (blood sugar) already in circulation in the bloodstream. If blood sugar is low — something which can happen normally whenever the kind or amount of food eaten is inadequate to support the degree of one's physical activity — the liver will turn loose stored glycogen, the raw material that in turn becomes glucose and is used for energy.

At this point, the alpha-2 cells of the pancreas are stimulated to store more glycogen, which scientists have identified as the controlling factor in balancing the production of another hormone, insulin, which regulates the metabolism of glucose and other carbohydrates.

Sounds complicated, doesn't it? What it means is that when you exercise you can simultaneously increase your expenditure of energy and stimulate the production of hormones that turn fat into more energy. The released energy, in turn, increases your blood flow, allowing your capillary network—the blood vessels supplying your muscles—to "breathe" better and work longer without tiring. Increased blood flow also carries away the waste material your muscles produce when they work—wastes that can result in stiff muscles.

This stimulation also makes your muscle fibers stronger and more efficient. For men, this means that the muscles will actually *grow*, since men have a sex hormone called testosterone that helps build muscle fiber. Women don't. That's why exercise will *not* produce hugely enlarged muscles in women. It *will* improve muscle tone. It's as simple as this: Muscles that are seldom used relax, then are torn down and used by the body for other functions. For example, a leg immobilized in a cast can lose up to five percent of its muscle in a week, and will certainly have lost its tone. But a muscle that is used regularly and properly increases its overall level of electrochemical activity and its tightness. That muscle will improve its tone.

If your muscles are in good shape and tone, they will perform a subsidiary role as a "corset" to hold your body in correct alignment—this is especially true with the muscles that support and move the back.

In that case, you'd think, the more exercise, the better.

That depends. It cannot be emphasized too strongly that random, or randomly chosen, exercise won't do. In fact, many sports—among them, weight-lifting or working with any kind of gymnastic apparatus, jogging, tennis, skiing, and even certain of the more vigorous forms of social dancing—can actually be harmful to your body if the movements called for are not performed correctly.

It's true that a program of rhythmic, repetitive activity like jogging, swimming, cycling, or rope jumping builds up your endurance and increases your capacity to absorb oxygen. But once you reach that capacity, no matter how hard you push your body, the heart and circulation can't deliver any more oxygen to the tissues, and you begin to approach exhaustion.

In addition, the fibers in your muscles "fire," just like cylinders in an engine, acting on signals from the nervous system. Not all the fibers in a given muscle fire every time you use it; instead, they spell each other: After six firings, a group of fibers starts to lose its ability to perform, and the stress is passed on to other fibers in the same muscle. If *all* the fibers in a muscle are overworked, the effort will be passed on to another muscle group. That's why, in order to work a muscle or muscle group thoroughly but without causing exhaustion and resulting stiffness, exercise must be both slow enough and repeated often enough to accomplish the desired result.

If you use the wrong muscles, even in walking, those muscles will eventually become strained and cause incorrect body alignment, pain, or both. The same thing happens when muscles are left unused.

The Nickolaus Technique concentrates on toning and exercising muscles—especially the ones not normally involved in our daily movements. This not only helps the body function more smoothly, but also primes the body for some of the more energetic physical activities it may not be able to sustain without preparation. And it even helps protect the body against such weaknesses of advancing age as lack of muscle resiliency, loss of skin tone, stiffness of the joints, and reduced energy. Streamlining your body and controlling its muscles preserves its vitality throughout life.

These exercises will not "pump up" your muscles as weight-lifting does—they were never intended to do that—but they will firm up your body, and prepare it for all kinds of other activity by improving strength, stamina, and flexibility, all the while developing your body into the useful instrument nature intended it to be. The exercises incorporate no machines or apparatus, but use the body itself for movement, resistance, and breathing control. They stress deep breathing action to supply the fuel—oxygen—that the muscles need to function effectively and that primes the circulatory system and prepares the body for joint movement by increasing flexibility and range of potential motion.

The movements of the Nickolaus Technique *cannot* be done in an unenergetic or offhand manner; they require effort and concentration. But they provide a tangible result with the greatest economy of time and effort—as little as two hours weekly is enough.

That is because the Technique takes into consideration the precise function of each muscle and the particular movements it must execute, as well as the whole physiology of body alignment, the way muscle fibers work, and how muscle groups interact with each other.

The exercises are performed in a set sequence. For example, they begin by loosening feet and ankles because that is necessary before you can get a good stretch through the legs—and limber legs are essential for doing some of the exercises that follow. In the same way, an exercise that works the lower back will be followed by one that stretches out the lower back and keeps it flexible.

Finally, and primarily, the exercises inte-grate body motion with regulated, directed breathing. As a result, you usually don't perspire heavily, you're not breathless, and the customary "day after" aches are virtually eliminated, because the constant pattern of breathing carries off the residue of the oxygen-production process that can cause muscle soreness.

Once you've mastered the exercises, some of the individual movements can be applied to specific problems arising from the generally pent-up, underexercised emotional and physical conditions we described in the last chapter—problems like tension, headache, back pain, and knee troubles. The exercises can be used at work during a break, or at home when you have a few minutes, as a means of relaxing and loosening yourself up. And, unlike many conventional forms of exercise, they *will* relax you, because they don't cause tension, fatigue, heavy perspiration and soreness.

Try the BREATHING (EXERCISE 1) described on page 47. It takes only a couple of minutes and can be a refreshing interlude—two or three times a day, if you want. You do need some floor space, but in a pinch a firm couch will do.

The HEAD ROLLS (EXERCISE 14) can be done while you're sitting at a desk or cross-legged on the floor—any floor. They are especially good for releasing the kind of tension that builds up in neck and shoulders during office or household chores, causing neck pain, headache, and stiffness. They feel good and can be used as a pick-me-up whenever needed.

The STANDING LEG AND BACK STRETCH (EXERCISE 29) and the STANDING LATERAL STRETCH (EXERCISE 28) both can be done in less than five minutes. They are excellent wake-up exercises and will increase your circulation while strengthening legs, back, and abdomen.

THE SQUEEZE (EXERCISE 27), during which you press your palms together while standing and tucking your pelvis under and tightening your buttocks, is another midday circulation exercise recommended for its refreshment value because it sends the blood racing through your system. In fact, it can be adapted to a sitting position and is a surefire remedy for "nodding out" at your desk: The shots of oxygen that it quickly delivers to your cells will help you to feel alert and energetic.

By such simple means you can begin to get in touch with your body and overcome the acquired feeling that exercise is somehow "unnatural."

Most Americans still have a sort of mental hangover from the nineteenth century, when the general attitude was that the less you knew about your body, the better. Today, many people still either ignore the body or treat it as an object separate from the mind. In fact, when it comes to overall physical conditioning, we are worse off than our Victorian ancestors. We accept as normal a degree of physical inadequacy that makes it impossible for our bodies to function joyfully, healthily, or even effectively. Too many Americans have simply abandoned their bodies, like someone moving out of a house.

The Nickolaus Technique recognizes the problem and acknowledges the body as the new frontier of our age. The Technique is based on a complete understanding of the body, and so, before proceeding with the exercises, we have devoted several chapters to describing in detail how your body functions, and how its functioning relates to what you do during the thirty sequenced exercises. Because that sort of understanding is the basis of the Nickolaus Technique.

The
Breath of
Life

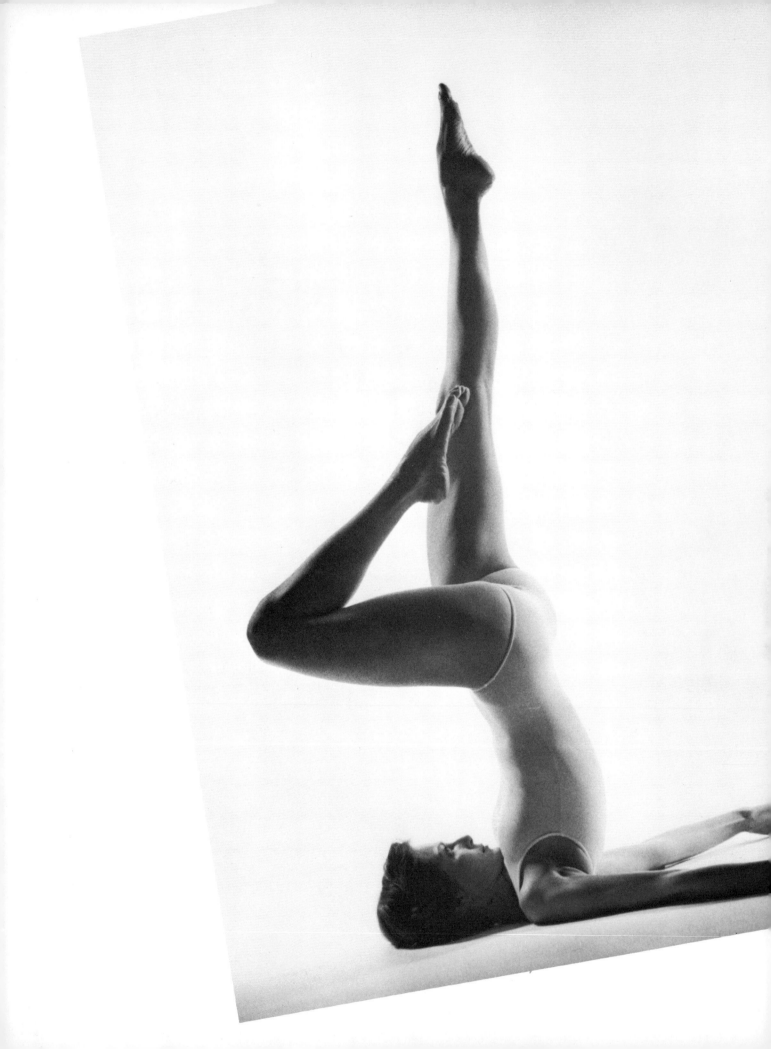

Breathing is the foundation of the Nickolaus Technique, as it is of life.

Surprisingly, most people don't really know *how* to breathe, though they do it all the time. Breathing is the way we get oxygen into our systems, and oxygen is essential for movement. Our muscles are "fired" by nervous impulses that are touched off by a variety of stimuli: emotion, the desire to perform some action, the urge to express something. If sufficient fuel—oxygen—isn't there when our muscles are fired, emotion will be restricted, action limited, and expressiveness stifled.

When your breathing is shallow or inefficient, the result is a kind of muscle and tissue starvation which can show up as aches, fatigue, depression, even insomnia. All parts of the body are affected by a shortage of oxygen, but because the tissues of the nervous system are especially sensitive to oxygen deficiency, it can have a profound impact not only on our bodies but also on our basic attitude toward life.

Depression—a feeling that afflicts more than eight million Americans every year— may be caused by the way you breathe, as Dr. Alexander Lowen, a pioneer of studies on mental states as they relate to body condition, observes in his book *Depression and the Body* (New York: Penguin Books, 1974):

"The relationship between depressed mood and depressed breathing is so direct and immediate that any technique which activates breathing loosens the grip of the depressive mood. It does so by actually increasing the body's energy level and by restoring some flow of bodily excitation."

There's a lot more to breathing than meets the eye — or even the mind's eye, unless you have trained body and mind together. Basically, what we loosely call "breathing" has an invisible and a (partially) visible function: internal respiration, the process by which the cells of your entire body trade carbon dioxide for fresh oxygen; and external breathing, the conscious process by which you draw oxygen into the bloodstream, by way of the lungs and expel carbon dioxide and water vapor — those wastes we mentioned earlier.

If the familiar inhale/exhale that is more or less under your direct control isn't working the way it should, you won't be drawing in sufficient oxygen to feed the cells of your body. Your muscles and mind won't be functioning as well as they can.

And unless you're actively doing something about it, that process *isn't* likely to be functioning as it should. We have been trained, largely by our environment, tension, and habit, to breathe in the upper part of our torsos. The next time you're in a department store, office, or other public place, sneak a look at the people there and see if you can spot the movement of their chests and stomachs as they breathe. If they are sitting or standing quite still and relaxed, you may notice that the stomach and lower chest area appear to move gently in rhythm with their breathing. If they are involved in heated conversation or frenzied activity, what you'll probably see is a lot of movement in the upper chest, little anywhere else.

That means breath doesn't reach the lower part of our lungs; the stale air and waste carbon dioxide that should be expelled on exhalation accumulate, so we're delivering a lot less oxygen into the bloodstream than our cells need to function at peak effectiveness. The result affects our skin tone, our muscles, and ultimately our morale.

A recent study suggests that one reason many people smoke cigarettes may be that they have an unconscious need to breathe deeply. Puffing a cigarette may allow them to take a deeper breath than when they inhale normally. Consequently, some smoking-avoidance clinics prescribe breathing exercises as an aid to overcoming the cigarette habit.

You might think people living in large cities would be better off *not* breathing deeply, considering the quality of what they're breathing. Actually, the opposite is true. Where there is air pollution, there's less healthful air in the lungs. They are forced to work harder to increase their capacity and deliver at least a reasonable proportion of usable fuel to the cells of the body.

Athletes, singers, actors, dancers, and others who lead active physical lives are forced by the nature of their work to acquire a technique of deep breathing; their bodies simply won't respond to the demands made on them unless sufficient oxygen is supplied through the lungs and the circulation.

The majority of us, unfortunately, have become separated from the very sensation of relaxed breathing — the way we breathe when we sleep. We have come to accept as normal a pattern of breathing that is shallow, tense, and, in fact, abnormal. We are stingy with our breath.

To correct this deficiency, we really have to return to basics and relearn the way we breathe.

First of all, we must understand that a principal muscle involved in the lungs' work is the diaphragm. It's a muscle we're hardly ever aware of, since it is inside the body — roughly speaking, it separates our chest cavity from our abdominal cavity — and it is only indirectly subject to voluntary control or exercise.

The diaphragm is a refinement peculiar to mammals. When the rib cage lifts, the dome-shaped diaphragm flattens out, further increasing the volume of the chest and causing air to rush into the lungs. When the rib cage presses downward, the diaphragm bulges upward — helping to squeeze out the air. (See illustration of BREATHING, EXERCISE 1.)

To achieve the degree of motion in the rib cage that lets the diaphragm do its work efficiently, we have to work on those areas that act as accessories to the diaphragm, specifically the abdominal muscles and the rib elevators or intercostals. Those muscles, properly developed, can produce significant increases in breathing effectiveness; however, their effect can be acquired only through voluntary control. For that reason, they require constant attention. In fact, your system is begging for it.

Without that attention — which can be focused only through a specialized exercise program built around correct breathing — it is only too easy to return to the "normal" pattern of shallow, upper-chest respiration that does not get oxygen where it needs to be in the amounts that are needed.

To experience the opposite of that pattern, lie on your back on a flat surface; the floor or a firm mattress will do. Place your hands lightly on your stomach. Imagine you are just drifting off to sleep. Let the air flow into your body, then gently expel it. You should become aware, on inhaling, of a low rise in your abdomen and lower stomach, a slight expansion in the muscles of your lower back. As you breathe out, there will be a gradual sinking of the lower stomach and abdomen, a relaxation of the lower back muscles.

The Nickolaus Technique aims at making this kind of breathing second nature, no matter what position your body is in, no matter what activity you are performing.

For, if we are likely to have trouble grasping the principles of correct breathing when the body is in repose, that trouble is compounded at times of stress or physical activity: At moments when we have to expend a lot of energy, whether physical or emotional, we tense up and lock our breath inside. In our western industrialized society, this is almost a reflex action.

Think of the last time you lifted a heavy object, or tugged at a stuck drawer, or were suddenly startled by a loud noise. Remember that feeling of tightness, of blood rushing to your face?

Nearly everyone reacts to sudden exertion by clutching up — sucking in the stomach when inhaling, and relaxing only when exhaling. But clutching up increases the effort you have to put out and makes it impossible to prepare for taking into the body the extra oxygen you need; if continued through a series of movements or a period of stress, it will wear you out quickly. What you should be doing, and what the Nickolaus Technique will show you *how* to do, is inhaling in preparation for a movement, and exhaling as you execute the movement.

If you've ever seen a weight lifter in action, you've probably noticed that when he is "jerking" a weight, he draws in his breath in a series of short puffs. But if he lifts a weight steadily, in a continuous movement, there is a slow, steady accumulation of breath at the same time. Well-trained dancers, too, breathe in rhythm with moments of exertion.

There is a reason for this: Coordinating deep abdominal breathing with moments of physical effort, as is done in the Nickolaus Technique, supplies a far greater quantity of oxygen to the system than it normally gets, helps the muscles to work more efficiently because they are well aerated, removes carbon dioxide residue that can interfere with muscle performance, and increases the lung capacity.

Deep breathing has an effect on muscles and organs other than those directly involved with the process of respiration. Besides expanding the lungs and letting the breathing muscles contract and then relax more completely, it also stimulates other trunk muscles, and consequently they relax more completely.

Furthermore, the effects of natural breathing on the mind can be downright startling. Some runners—and even weekend joggers—notice that when they are forced into a more natural and rhythmic pattern of breathing, they experience a "rush": Their senses become sharper and thought processes more acute. Students of the Nickolaus Technique have reported similar results—the increased flow of energy (oxygen) to the brain and the stimulation of circulation seem to make for a lively mind in a lively body.

The effectiveness of all the exercises in the Technique depends on proper, natural breathing. It is an indispensable warm-up. More, it is a "second exercise" that goes on simultaneously with every movement. Indeed, it might be better described as the primary exercise that supports all the others.

It is for this reason that we deal with breathing here, before the detailed description of the Nickolaus Technique. It is so important, there is no point in proceeding until you have mastered it.

Turn to page 47 and read the description of the first exercise in the Technique. Before you even begin any of the other exercises, it's a good idea to practice this kind of breathing until it's second nature to you at every moment of the day, whether you're sitting, standing, running, walking, or whatever.

As an exercise, by itself, it will go a long way toward improving your energy, physical condition, and general attitude toward life.

Foot to Knee to Hip

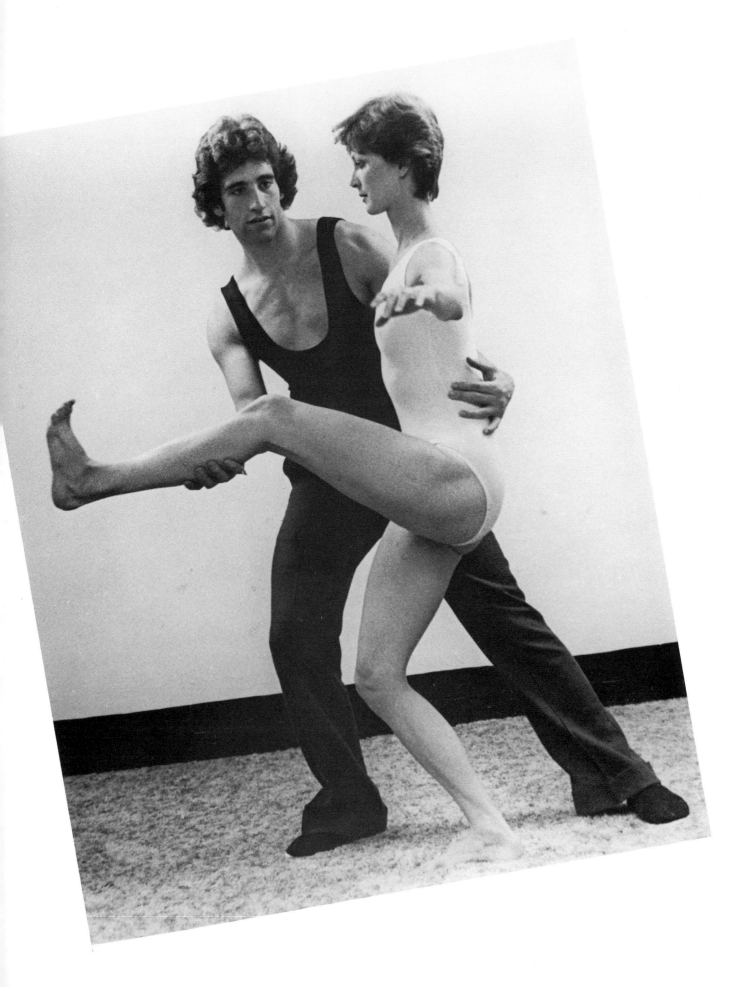

"The more one studies man's ability to stand and to walk, the more remarkable these acts seem. We do not really stand on our feet the way a lamp stands on its base; what we do is balance on a collection of small, movable and loosely connected bones, only three of which touch the ground." So says Fritz Kahn, M.D., in *The Human Body* (New York: Random House, 1965); and indeed our coordination, our stamina, our entire physical and mental health depend to a large extent on establishing a correct and often delicate balance between ankle, knee, and hip. It is recognition of this relationship that helps make the Nickolaus Technique what it is—an invaluable tool for getting in touch with your body. If you want to get the most out of the Technique, it's important that you understand the crucial elements in that balance.

THE FOOT

Because the foot is the extremity farthest from both the heart and the eyes, it is the limb from which we can most easily become "disconnected." This lack of communication often permits us to do things to our own feet that would be grounds for criminal action if someone else did them to us.

We cram them into shoes that are too tight, chafe them in shoes that are too loose, let them wobble around on platform shoes or stiletto heels, and in general treat them like cast-off objects rather than what they are: the foundation of our body's motion.

Whether we realize it or not, the condition of the foot has a very direct effect on other parts of the body. The sciatic nerve, for example, connects to the spinal column, running down the back of the leg into the foot. If the metatarsal arch presses on the endings of the sciatic nerve, the result can be lower back pain. Postural problems originating in the foot can also cause sore knees, aching leg muscles, stiff neck, and headache.

But the most common effect of standing improperly is backache. For instance, if you stand with your weight on your heels — a frequent error and one that is practically forced on people by the newly popular shoes that feature sunken heels — the arching of the lumbar areas of the spine to compensate for this stance will fatigue the spinal muscles. The resulting lack of alignment will then put a strain on ligaments, tendons, and working parts of the joints. Long-term result: a whole range of orthopedic problems over an extended period of time.

So let us consider the foot. The first thing to look at is the shoe you put it in. Choosing footwear exclusively for reasons of fashion is like choosing a home because it has a flashy facade. From a physiological standpoint, the high heel is the single most destructive factor in foot damage. What features should a good shoe have? Here are some suggestions:

— It should be long enough so the end of the great toe is not against the end of the shoe, but not so long that the foot slides forward from the heel upper.

— The front must be wide enough not to cramp the toes, but snug enough so the forefoot won't slide about. The heel must be held snugly both at the sides and behind.

— It should have enough height over the instep so the instep isn't pushed downward.

— The lines of the shoe must correspond to the lines of the foot.

— The shank fit is most important. If the whole sole of the foot is utilized as the weight-bearing surface, it will be easier to carry the distributed load. That means you should choose a shoe whose shank fits your individual arch.

— If a woman *must* wear a heel, she should wear one no higher than two inches, with a broad base. This will tend to throw the weight forward and keep it off the heel.

If you want to know whether you're walking correctly, take a look at the heel of your shoe; it should be worn at the outside center. A heel that's worn too much on the outside of your foot means you're walking pigeon-toed. If it's worn on the inside, watch out for real trouble. This indicates your middle foot bone is sinking, or sunken. The resulting toed-out, Charlie Chaplin walk might seem cute, but there won't be anything cute about the complications (back pain is only one possibility) that are apt to accompany it.

If we seem to be giving you nothing but bad news about your feet, there is one overriding piece of good news: We start with nature on our side. The foot we are given at birth is a marvel of construction. It is built like a bridge, with the heel as apex and the span of the metatarsal arch stretching just above the toes, from big toe to little.

That construction allows the foot that's kept in good condition to act as a shock absorber for walking and running, jumping and landing. Ideally, the body's weight should rest on those three points, so that the body is poised for movement.

The skeleton of the foot has three divisions: the tarsis — seven bones that form the ankle area; the metatarsis — five bones of the middle foot; and the phalanges — fourteen bones.

When any of those bones moves, there has to be a muscle to move it. Since most bones move at least two ways, several groups of muscles can be involved in what seems a simple movement. The stronger the muscles, the stronger the support. That is why it's so essential to strengthen the foot through exercise.

And jogging or running around a tennis court is not necessarily going to exercise your feet in a way that strengthens them. In fact, if your body weight is distributed incorrectly because of sloppy posture or weak muscles, tennis or running may tend to further weaken your feet, or may even strain the delicate connections of bone and tissue. The only way to build strong feet or correct common foot problems is through exercises specifically designed for the foot.

That's why, in all of the movements in the Nickolaus Technique, the foot is in a specific position — most often, flexed — so that it is being continually exercised.

The initial exercises in the Technique, after breathing, involve the foot. This is, first, because we are so out of touch with our feet. It is urgent that we become aware of how we hold and use them during the entire program of movements — and, ultimately, at every moment of our lives.

Then, too, exercising the foot increases circulation and relaxes and tones the muscles in the foot. Working on the feet at the beginning of the program assures a rush of blood to these areas, supplying the needed fuel to carry off the by-products of circulation, and works out any tension, preparing the foot for everything that follows.

THE KNEE

The knee is the largest joint in our bodies, and it provides an excellent example of the intimate relationship between correct skeletal alignment, good muscle tone, and total physical well-being.

It supplies, to a large extent, our potential for motion. It transports us through life — bending, bouncing, bounding, bicycling. The driving action of the knee with its constant cycle of pistonlike movements allows us to walk, run, and jump. Its movement involves gliding and rotation, which are more complicated processes than the easy, hingelike working of the other major joints.

Picture the knee's position in your body. Below it is the heel section with its two axle-like bones, one above the other, on which balances a pair of columnlike bones that reach to the knee. The loose knee joint rests on that combination, and on it rest the thigh bones and the entire body.

Despite its size and position of responsibility, the knee is a delicate and temperamental instrument. Many physicians regard it as one of nature's mistakes, because it is basically unstable.

Celia Sparger, who was for years consulting physiotherapist to the Royal Ballet School, says the knees are "second only to the feet as a source of trouble. They are vulnerable and unforgiving joints. An ankle will recover from quite severe injury with no aftereffects, but the knee has a long memory, and any real damage to it can be a major calamity."

Why is the knee so subject to injury?

Because, as we've already suggested, though at first it appears hingelike, it has, when in a semiflexed position, the potential for lateral movement — in other words, it can be moved, or can slip, sideways, possibly beyond the range within which movement can be sustained safely. That condition, combined with the knee's high proportion of cartilage and ligaments in comparison with other joints, makes it a particularly easy target for strains and torn cartilage or ligaments.

Significantly, Dr. Sparger stresses that "a knee which is in good alignment rarely gives any trouble."

Injury occurs around a joint when the range of motion is taken beyond the capabilities of the muscles to protect tendons, cartilage, and ligaments. Because of the close relationship between muscles and the cartilage, ligaments, and tendons involved in a joint's movement, it will be more difficult to injure your knee when the muscles are strong enough to hold it in the correct alignment.

Two massive columns of bone — the thigh and the shin bones — are connected at your kneecap by a network of tendons and ligaments that draw their power from the massive muscles extending from your knee joint in all directions. Only by strengthening those muscles can you protect the delicate machinery of the knee and keep it properly aligned.

You can understand the function of your knee in terms of the general observation that movement is a matter of action and reaction: You bend the knee to take a step, straighten it, then bend it again to take another step. And all the while, the knee is acting as a spring that takes all the weight of your body.

To support that constant cycle of motion, the muscles around your knee need to be strong, flexible, and well supplied with oxygen. To maintain the necessary balance between bending and straightening, they must be trained to "feel" maximum bend and maximum extension.

In the Nickolaus Technique, the LEG LIFTS (EXERCISE 18) can be considered a knee exercise, in addition to their obvious benefit to the thighs and abdomen. As your thigh muscles are strengthened, the movement of the knee joint also becomes cleaner and more powerful. What's more, if the lifts are done correctly, with the leg stretching *out* as you lift it, they will stretch and strengthen the muscles on either side of the knee. Finally, the exercise will increase the flow of blood and, therefore, oxygen to the whole leg area.

EXERCISES 4 and 5, the SINGLE LEG STRETCH and DOUBLE LEG STRETCH, which work the knee first at maximum flexion and then at maximum extension, develop flexibility and a feeling for what your knee can do when it is correctly aligned with the rest of the leg.

Like other exercises in the Technique, these movements coordinate thought, breathing, and body movement and awareness. It is unimaginable that anyone could, through an act of will, align the intricate mechanism of the knee so that it would never be in danger of injury. But through repeating these exercises, the muscles of your leg will "learn" what correct alignment feels like.

At the same time, the danger of carrying your knee beyond the safe range of motion will be minimized, because that safe range of motion will be considerably extended.

One student who had been taking the Nickolaus Technique for several months commented, "I feel so secure about my legs and knees. They've become so strong, and I've become so conscious of what they're doing, I don't think I could injure them if I wanted to."

THE HIP

The hip — and the pelvis, the socket into which the hip is plugged — is as dependable as the knees are fluky; and a good thing, too, considering its central position in the body.

The hip is the axis on which your body rotates. Each hip joint supports half the body weight above the pelvis; it is involved in shifting weight; it is responsible for movement.

But in itself it does not move as much as you might expect. Its socket is deep and surrounded by large ligaments. These supporting ligaments are so numerous and heavy that they serve to limit motion more than to secure the joint. If normal, the joint is rarely dislocated.

Dr. Sparger of the Royal Ballet, who had such discouraging things to say about the knee in the last section, has a solid vote of confidence for the hip. She says that among dancers, "the hip joint as such is peculiarly free from trouble."

That doesn't mean the hip can be left to its own devices, so to speak. It may be relatively free from trouble, but — at least, for anyone leading an active life — the muscles around it are not.

In sports, this is particularly true. The violent exertion, the gravitational load, and the abrupt changes in direction required in athletics make the muscles of the hip especially susceptible to injury. And if the hip itself is stiff and inflexible, the muscles that lead out of it — particularly the leg muscles — will be correspondingly limited in their range and their energy.

When the hip is injured, it is often slow to heal, and the damage tends to recur. We can learn a lot from athletes and dancers, who prevent such injuries by slow, careful stretching of the hip muscles before engaging in activity.

As we've pointed out, because the muscles in the hip area serve to limit motion rather than to secure the joint, it is necessary to work on them to achieve the flexibility and range of movement this section of your body should have to permit easy, coordinated mo-

tion. In compensating for a hip joint that's not as flexible as it should be, we often put undue strain on the knee. So solving or preventing hip problems also reduces problems of the knee.

Often, the halting movement associated with old age results from weakness or partial atrophy of the muscles that control the hip, and the resulting involvement of the knee joint. In most cases, this condition is not due so much to illness or anything basic to the nature of aging as it is to lack of use. Sedentary people, in particular, are likely to have hips years older than the chronological age of their bodies.

This is why it's important for you to work on the muscles around the hip joint. It's not just because you want a slender, taut hip line. This versatile ball-and-socket joint is the director of movement. It has a wide range of motion and the capacity to send you wherever you want to go: forward, backward, sideways. It even allows you to cross your legs.

Many of the exercises in the Nickolaus Technique work the muscles of the abdomen, legs, and buttocks, crucial in gaining control and increased range in movements involving the hips. Of special importance, however, is the SMALL BRIDGE (EXERCISE 8), which works the entire pelvic area and strengthens the buttock muscles at the same time that it stretches the hip joint. You can see the results of this series of movements in the picture illustrating PERFECT POSTURE (EXERCISE 30).

One of the reasons the Nickolaus Technique affects your body with unusual speed and completeness is that, while each of the exercises is designed to broaden one range of motion or work one area of the body, if you perform them correctly you are simultaneously exercising the rest of your body.

LEG LIFTS, for example, are specifically for

the development of the thigh — but when you sit on the floor with your head erect, chest high, and abdominal muscles pulled in, you are exercising all the other areas of your body.

You will also realize a total sense of strength and control from the pelvic movement and flexibility the exercises develop.

The
Spine

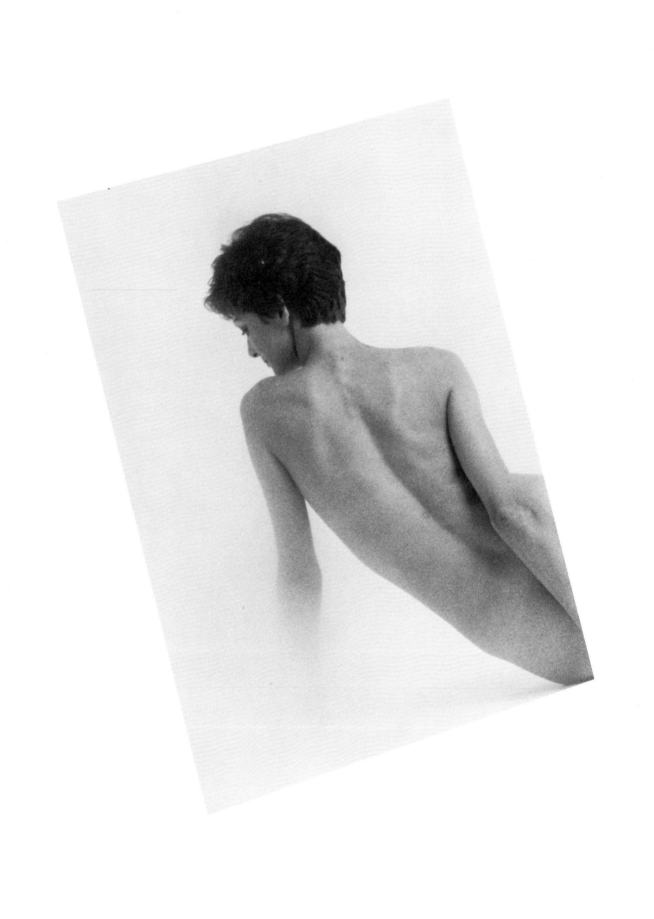

No area of the body demonstrates more dramatically than the spine the interdependence of mind, physical fitness, and the enjoyment of life.

In a sense, the spine is the root of our life: The oldest part of our body, in terms of evolution, it comes down to us directly from the notochord, the rodlike cord of cells found in the lower forms of amphibious life from which we are descended.

But no amphioxus or cyclostome ever had the trouble with its notochord that we have with our spines — or, to be more accurate, our backs. It is tempting to guess that when the first human being stood up, the first backache struck.

The very way we describe our backs suggests how little we understand them. We talk about them as if they were rods of reinforced steel: "the back*bone* . . . the spinal *column*."

Nothing could be further from the actuality. The spine is neither a bone nor a column: It is an S-shaped line of bones, with disks in between for cushioning, and with ligaments holding the bones and disks — which they do rather loosely.

Ideally, a support column is firm and inflexible. In the human spine, nature has sacrificed rigidity in order to secure a relatively wide range of movement. The result of this attempt to combine two incompatible qualities is an unstable structure which may be seriously damaged by sports as diverse as golf and weight-lifting. Often, these injuries are painful, slow to heal, and quick to recur.

To understand the scope of the problem, consider this: At a conservative estimate, seven million Americans are under treatment for some form of back malady every day of the year. The latest figures from the National Health Survey show that each year Americans make approximately nineteen million visits to doctors to complain of backache — a problem reported more frequently than headache, fatigue, or even the common cold.

The remarkable thing is that, out of the almost endless potential for discomfort and injury the structure of the spine presents, the overwhelming majority of back problems stem from a single basic cause. Significantly, that cause is not found in the spine itself.

A combined medical group from New York University and Columbia University conducted a study covering 5000 consecutive patients with back pain. Because the study included every back-pain patient seen at the two universities until the total of 5000 was reached, it represented an unselected sample. Its results apply to everyone with back pain, rather than to a special segment of back-pain patients.

The central problem was not "slipped" disks, arthritis, tumor, or, in fact, any disease or malfunction of the back itself. In more than four out of five cases, backache was related to muscular insufficiency or inadequate flexibility of muscles and tendons.

If it is clear that in the majority of cases the prime cause of backache is muscular inadequacy, it is even clearer that one set of mus-

cles in particular is more often responsible than any other. And those muscles are not in the back.

What makes it possible for people to lift weights that otherwise could break the spine is a rigid abdominal cavity and a firm structure of stomach muscles. Even in the most ordinary movements, strong abdominal muscles keep the stomach from sagging forward. The forward sag is what imposes dangerous stresses on the lower, or lumbar, region of the spine.

When the abdominal muscles are flabby, the weight of the abdominal contents is thrown forward, tending to pull the spine with it — in chronic backache patients, abdominal muscles are often less than *one-third* as strong as back muscles. (Ideally, both sets of muscles should be equally strong.)

Strangely, that is good news. For what it indicates is that a clear majority of patients with back pain (more than four in five, according to the New York study) are not suffering from organic spinal disorder — at least, that it is not the cause of their pain — nor do they require surgery.

What's more, the recurrence of back pain in those cases can be reduced in frequency or severity or both, and may even be eliminated, by simple corrective measures.

It is precisely those corrective measures that are an integral part of the Nickolaus Technique.

But before we explain how and why that is true, let's take a closer look at the way the back functions.

The unstable "column" of the spine is held together by tough, fibrous ligaments; but these by themselves cannot support the spine, give it balance, or allow it to move. For those tasks, some 140 muscles are necessary.

At times, they are no light tasks. Take a man who weighs 180 pounds: When he bends forward so his trunk is flexed 60 degrees from the vertical, the muscle force required to keep him from falling is 450 pounds. Add a 50-pound weight (a heavy suitcase, two large bags of groceries), and in the same position the required muscle force will be 750 pounds. At the same time, there will be a compression force of about 850 pounds put on the fifth lumbar vertebra — the last movable bone at the bottom of the spine.

Inevitably, if the muscles supporting your back are even slightly out of condition, you are inviting discomfort, if not disaster.

Equally important, those 140-odd muscles protect the spine with their bulk. Strong back-support muscles can even compensate to a considerable extent for injury to other parts of the spinal structure — some Nickolaus students have been able, in spite of severely damaged spines, to lead normal lives, virtually free of pain, by building up the musculature that protects and supports the spine.

Much of the trouble with our backs begins in our heads. People who are uptight, socially rigid, or just plain scared — conditions that are not uncommon in the twentieth century — tend to have tight, inflexible backs. In the case of those who hold back emotion, the main tensions are often found in the long muscles of the body, especially those along the spinal column.

Even if you are emotionally free as a bird, you may have difficulty keeping the muscles of your back in good working order if you don't know what a correctly functioning back feels like — as you will know if you do EXERCISE 8 (SMALL BRIDGE) or EXERCISE 30 (PERFECT POSTURE).

As we have said, flabby abdominal muscles often result in greater or lesser damage to the back. When belly muscles are not tight, the resulting "swayback" posture does to the spine, in a sense, what being immobilized in a cast does to the muscles of a person who has broken a leg. Connective tissues have a tendency to contract rapidly if they are not used; and when the cast is removed, the person may experience stiffness of the knee — even though the knee was not involved in the original injury — and require a program of exercise to restore flexibility.

When weak abdominal muscles cause forward curvature of the spine, the connective tissues in the back of the spine shorten, while those in front are stretched. If that situation is allowed to continue, the mobility of the spine can be considerably reduced. Eventually, even "fusing" of the vertebrae can result.

There is, however, a positive aspect to the prevalence of weak abdominal muscles as a source of back trouble: Correct exercise of the abdominal muscles is often all that is necessary to eliminate backache, and the Nickolaus Technique places special emphasis on this problem area. Since each exercise is based on a breathing pattern, the lower abdominal muscles are constantly contracting and expanding. The lower intestinal tract is pushed against the lumbar area of the spine, and becomes nature's "girdle." In this way, the lower back muscles, and the entire back, are protected from strain.

That process is reinforced by the importance, in so many of the exercises, of a strong abdominal contraction as preparation for movement in other parts of the body.

This reinforcement, from one exercise to another, is basic to the Nickolaus Technique. Furthermore, once you learn what a correct abdominal contraction feels like, you carry it not only through all the movements of the Technique, but also through the actions you perform in your daily life.

In effect, your body learns to exercise itself.

How to Use This Book

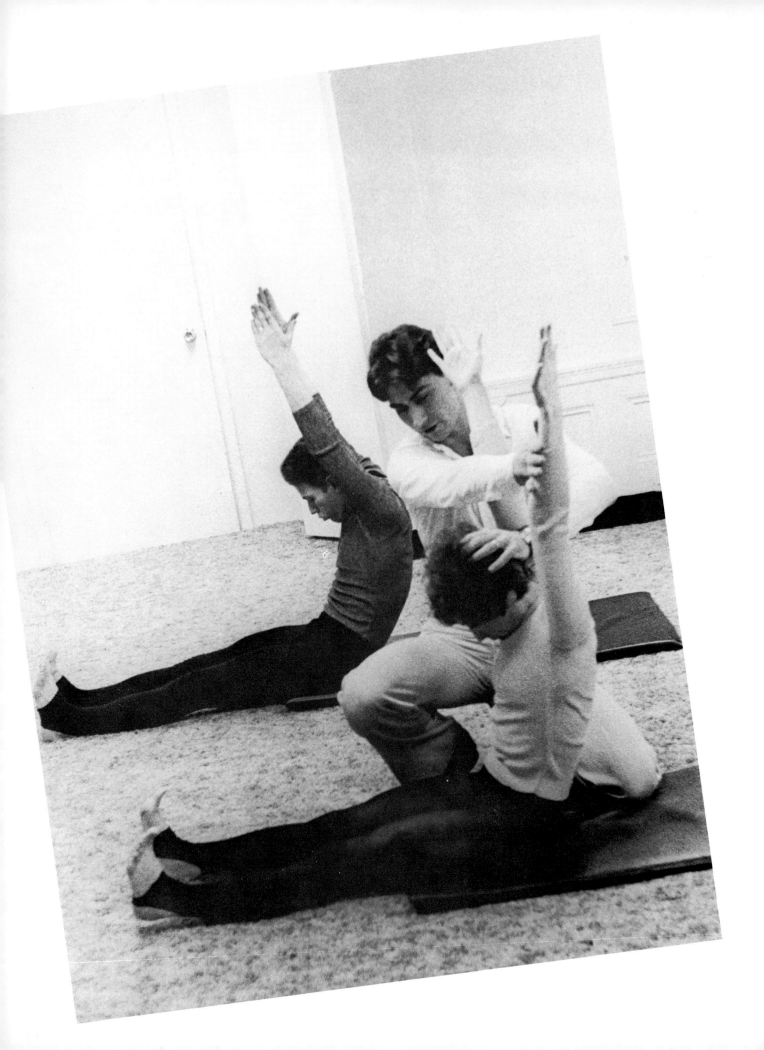

Since the Nickolaus Technique has been planned as a sequence of thirty exercises supported by the pulses of rhythm and breathing, the target to aim for is to be able to do the exercises with a "through" line from beginning to end, without skipping the two rest periods, but without pausing as you make the transition from one movement to another.

It isn't easy, though with effort it can become pleasurable — especially as you begin to see the results. But in the beginning you will have to work to master each individual position before you can move easily from one to another. The Nickolaus Technique is a lifetime program; it is vital to take the time to get each position right, since there is a reason for each of them.

At the same time, remember that doing all the exercises briskly, in the correct sequence, *is* the target. It is that sequence that makes the Nickolaus Technique unique. Many of the individual movements and positions are found in other disciplines — yoga, dance exercises, gymnastics. But this particular progression and rhythm are found nowhere outside the Nickolaus Technique.

It builds from simple warm-up movements to exercises that require increasing amounts of energy and concentration, and back down to movements that, in effect, restate what the body has learned and send you from the exercise mat to your home or office, onto the tennis court, ski slopes, or wherever, with a growing sense of balance and control. In fact, just studying the logic behind the arrangement of the exercises will teach you something about your body.

The point of the coordinated pattern of breathing and contraction that threads through all the individual movements of the Nickolaus Technique is to get the body and mind relating to each other.

At first, it will seem difficult in many of the exercises to get breathing and movement coordinated. The more you do them, the more your body will become unified.

For example, in the FOOT FLEX (EXERCISE 3, page 52) your feet are working in a four-count against the steady, slow two-count of the breath. At first, this may take some concentration; but after a few days you will find the two elements support each other easily and naturally and become a whole.

It will also take some concentration in the beginning to master the abdominal contraction which, in so many of the exercises, accompanies the expulsion of breath and prepares for the start of the movement. In every case, this contraction is the most essential part of the movement; it should start at the pubic bone and work all the way up. It should always occur in the lower abdominals, not in the rib cage.

Both those principles — steadiness of breathing and rhythmic contraction — work together with each other and with each of the exercises.

The question is bound to arise in your mind: How will I really know if I'm doing the exercises correctly?

Without an instructor, it can be extremely difficult.

Now, pause a moment before you hurl this book across the room. In the first place, studying the exercises and grasping the principles behind them will give you a more complete sense of how your body functions and moves.

What's more, there is tremendous value to be gained from working on the exercises by yourself, in your home. Ideally, this book should be used as an educational tool to help you understand your body, as a helpful supplement to class work.

Of course, there's no comparison between learning on your own and having the assistance of an instructor trained to teach the Technique. Not to mention the inevitable problems of motivation when there's no one but yourself to encourage you to persist. But suppose this book is your first introduction to the Nickolaus Technique and, for the time being, your only contact with the exercises. How can you use it?

To begin with, slowly. Before you attempt a single exercise, read through the whole Technique one exercise at a time, checking the pictures and trying to visualize your body going through the movements. Then go through the whole sequence again, this time trying to see how each exercise flows into the next. Do this several times, until you have a real picture in your mind of the entire series as an integrated and connected whole.

In a sense, you should finally think of the entire Nickolaus Technique as a single long exercise, lasting approximately an hour. When you can do it with that tempo and continuity, it will get your heart working faster and your circulation moving more briskly, in addition to all its other benefits.

But again we stress, slow and easy does it. Don't try to tackle the whole thing at once. The best approach is to take EXERCISES 1 through 5 and work on them slowly until you can do them without interruption. This alone will probably take several sessions. Then, after repeating the first five, go on to EXERCISES 6 through 10, approaching them in the same way.

Any exercise that causes the slightest strain or discomfort should be eliminated until you can consult someone experienced in the Technique. However, on one score you can set your mind at rest: It's virtually impossible to injure yourself doing the Nickolaus Technique—*provided you pay strict attention to the warning that accompanies EXERCISES 16 (THE BIRD) and 20 (THE BOW).*

That statement requires some qualification. You *can* hurt yourself just walking down the street, if your body is out of shape and/or you don't understand it—one reason we so strongly emphasize the value of instruction. But these exercises are designed to minimize the chances of self-injury. It is difficult to overstretch a muscle if you're not pulling on or against something outside your body. None of these movements involves pulling on another object, and very few of them even work one set of muscles against another—much less dangerous, in any case, since your muscles are unlikely to pull against each other to the point where they are injured.

Nevertheless, an important warning: Do not undertake this or any other exercise program, especially on your own, without first consulting your doctor. The Nickolaus Technique was developed under medical supervision and has been endorsed by doctors, but no one except your own physician can assure you that you can perform these movements without danger of injury. If you have been extremely sedentary before embarking on this program, go slowly and don't push yourself.

Under no circumstances work on the exercises out of sequence, for that will considerably reduce their effect. It's all right, as we've indicated, to take a given sequence of exercises and concentrate on them; but don't, for example, jump from EXERCISE 2 to EXERCISE 15.

You can also "excerpt" specific exercises for specific problems. The opening warm-up (BREATHING, FOOT CIRCLES, FOOT FLEX, SINGLE LEG STRETCH) is, by itself, an excellent corrective for the most common physical problem, weak abdominal muscles.

Another caution, however: "Spot" exercise alone is at worst harmful and at best of limited effectiveness. You cannot really correct deficiencies in isolated joints or muscle groups without exercising *all* joints, *all* muscle groups, because of the body's delicately balanced interdependence. A key point of the Nickolaus Technique is that it recognizes that interdependence and views the body as a connected whole.

It might be more fun and also more effective to enlist the participation of a friend or spouse in learning the exercises. It's not always easy to get through a sequence if you have to keep turning back to the book to remind yourself what comes next. With a partner, each of you can take turns reading the other through exercises and checking positions against those in the illustrations.

If you decide you're going to try the exercises, make it a real commitment. Set aside a couple of hours a week—in the morning, after you get home from work, before you go to bed, while the laundry's in the washer or the dinner's cooking—and make those hours your time with the Nickolaus Technique.

Find a mat, a rug, or a section of the carpet—*not* a bed; it's too soft. Take the phone off the hook; put on some relaxing music, or just lie down and listen to the quiet. Turn off any harsh lights. Relax. Unwind.

If you're doing the exercises alone, keep the book by you, close at hand, so you don't have to keep dashing across the room to double-check a position. Just before you settle down and relax, read once more through the exercises you're going to work on.

Wear comfortable clothes, and as few of them as possible — underwear or gym shorts for men, perhaps leotards for women. In fact, if you're by yourself, naked is best. Certainly, avoid belts, shoes, or anything that might restrict movement.

Okay. In your mind's eye have you got yourself relaxed, comfortable, unwound? Then you're ready to turn the page and discover the Nickolaus Technique.

The Nickolaus Technique

THE EXERCISES

1 Lie on a rug or mat with your knees bent enough to keep your lower back against the floor. Knees and feet are about eight inches apart. The shoulders, hips, knees, and ankles should be aligned, as in the picture. Keep your feet on the floor with toes turned slightly inward so the arches are lifted. Let your shoulders relax so they are resting against the floor. Your chin should be toward your chest, your mouth slightly open. Try to press the back of your neck against the floor. This is your basic breathing position.

EXERCISE 1* BREATHING

The lung is like a sponge; the point is to fill it as full as possible, then squeeze all the air out. Impurities settle in the bottom of the lung; exercising it forces them out. By helping you to a growing awareness of how your breathing functions, this exercise will help you to control your breath, increase lung capacity, and break up any congestion that has accumulated in your lungs as a result of air pollution or excessive smoking. In addition, deep breathing relaxes you and prepares you for the exercises that follow. In fact, it's good preparation for just about any physical activity, from tennis to walking.

*Exercises marked with an asterisk are recommended for the warm-up described on page 140.

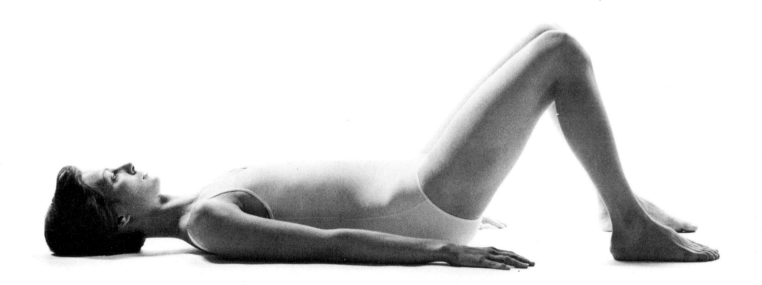

2 Relax. Imagine you're lying in bed, just before drifting off, and let everything go. Every muscle in your body should be loose. Place your hands on your stomach with the middle fingers meeting at the navel so that you can feel the movement of your abdominal muscles.

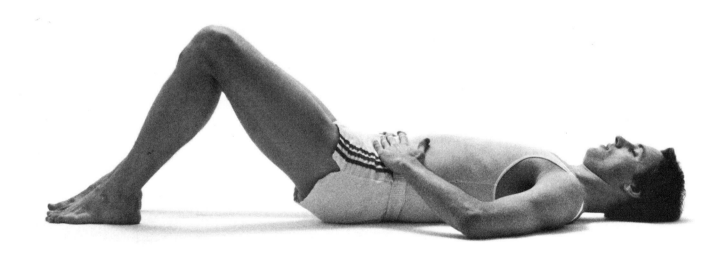

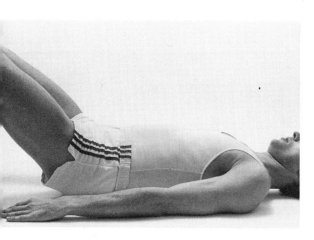

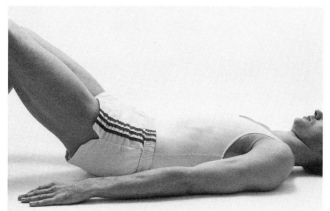

3 Inhale on a slow count of four, letting the diaphragm descend (actually, in this position, you have almost no choice) and with your fingers feel your abdomen expand and rise. (In the photograph the hands are *not* resting on the stomach — so you can see what happens more clearly.) Let the breath flow upward into the chest, expanding the upper part of the torso, too.

4 Now allow the breath to flow out of you, gently contracting first the muscles of the chest, then those of the abdomen, until the air is spent. With the abdominal contraction, feel the lower part of your back make solid contact with the floor — it's a kind of mini-"bump." Again, a slow count of four.

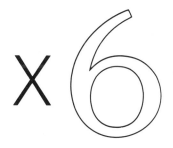

Do the exercise six times.

It is important to maintain an even flow of breath, with no jerking between inhale and exhale. Steps 1 through 4 should be performed in a steady, continuous rhythm — don't separate the different phases of your breathing. There should be no tension, except in the abdomen, when breathing out.

EXERCISE 2*

FOOT CIRCLES

A common factor in foot sprains is that the sideways motions of the ankles have seldom been used, so their strength and flexibility are diminished. This exercise, by developing strength and flexibility, helps to prevent strains and to increase the range of motion. It also works the muscle over the shinbone, reducing the chances of a "shin splint," the tenderness that can develop along the front of the lower leg after hard running, or walking on hard surfaces like pavement.

1 Starting in the previous position, bring right knee to the chest, left hand resting on the knee and right hand near ankle; elbows are slightly raised. Your foot is flexed, with the toes pulled toward the knee. Pay special attention to the big toe, since it will tend to lead the others.

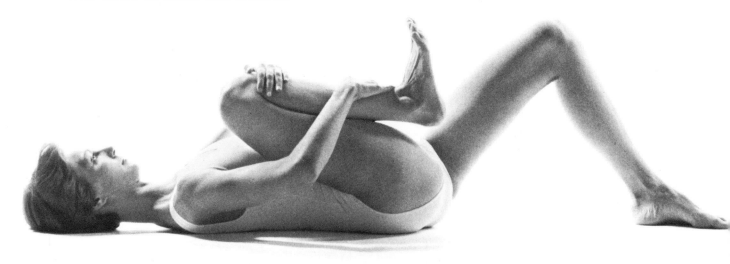

2 As you inhale, circle the foot clockwise until the toe is pointed away from you; then exhale as you continue the circle to the starting position, when your foot is flexed again. Make five clockwise circles; then reverse and circle the foot in a counter-clockwise direction five times.

Repeat with the other foot.

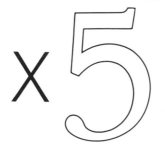

X5 Do this exercise five times with each foot.

You should feel a good, vigorous stretch across the top of the ankle and on the sides of the foot as you make a steady, continuous circle with no interruption in your movement or your breathing. You may notice that your shins feel pulled, almost achy, as you do this exercise. That's because the muscles you're working — those that support the ankle and shin — almost never get any exercise. That achy feeling shouldn't persist after you've been doing the exercise for a few weeks. Avoid any movement in the knee joint or any halting as you make the circle. It isn't easy at first to synchronize breathing with the movement of the foot. Don't worry; with time and determination, it will come.

EXERCISE **3**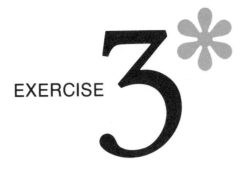 FOOT FLEX

This intensifies the effect of the last exercise and works the calf more, firming it up. It also tones up the metatarsal, which is lifted as the toes are pointed. Both this and the last exercise aid in developing coordination — as, indeed, do all the exercises in the Technique.

1 Still in the same position, pull one knee to the chest and grasp it, elbows up. The foot is flexed, toes pulled back toward the knee. The other foot rests on the floor; the knee is bent, the toes turned slightly inward.

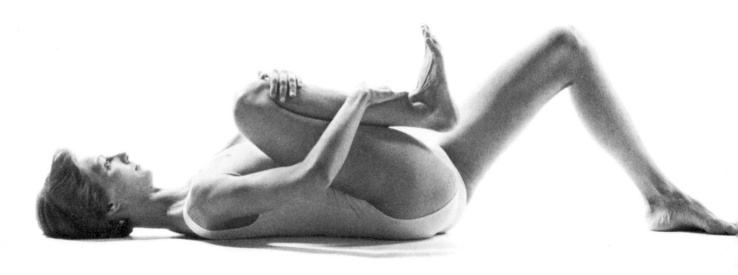

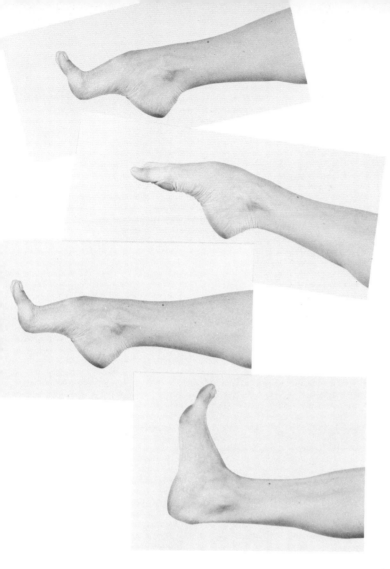

2 During inhalation, first arch the foot, extending the metatarsal but keeping the toes flexed back; then point the toes. Then exhale, bringing *just* the toes up, *then* flexing the foot — again, two separate and distinct motions, though they should flow into each other. There should be a stretch and contraction across the top of the ankle, a distinct passage from arch to point and back again.

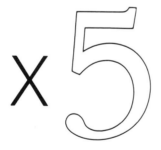

Do the exercise five times for each foot.

You may find it difficult to get a good stretch in your foot at first because the muscles are so underused. You may also find that extending the metatarsal and pointing the toe hard causes a cramp in your foot. This happens because circulation in your foot is poor — something the Technique can correct in time. For now, if your foot cramps, relax it a little; then go on with the exercise.

EXERCISE **4** *

SINGLE LEG
STRETCH

This exercise is a great muscle toner. Stretching promotes muscle tone, and this movement stretches and strengthens three areas of the body. The motion of pulling the knee down to the chest stretches the groin and prepares the hamstrings for EXERCISE 6.

The reach contracts the lower and upper abdominal muscles and—if done properly—the buttocks and seat muscles, and it stretches the muscles in the neck and shoulders.

1 Start in the basic breathing position. Draw your left knee down toward the chest, with left hand grasping the ankle and right hand on your knee. Keep your foot flexed at all times. When you breathe in, bring your knee down as far as you can, pulling toward the armpit. Your heel should be pulled toward the back of your thigh. Keep the tip of your spine on the floor and hips as square as possible.

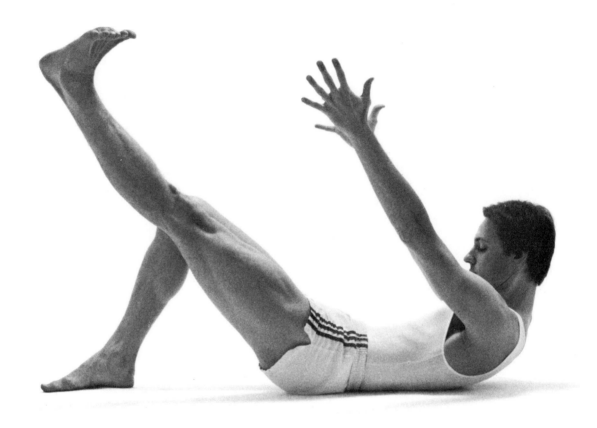

2 Lift your head up, contract the abdominal muscles, and breathe out. As you exhale, extend your leg until it is straight and parallel with the thigh of the bent leg. At the same time, extend your arms, palms facing each other, parallel to the stretched leg. Lower back remains on floor.

3 Inhale and come back to original position.

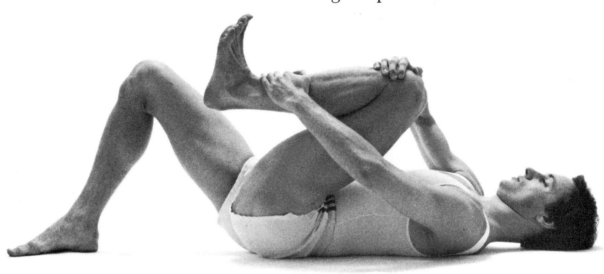

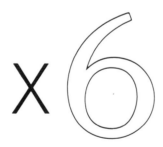

Do the exercise six times with each leg.

Do not allow either hip to come off the floor more than the other one, as will happen if you use the foot of your bent leg to brace yourself and push up, rather than pulling with your stomach muscles to raise your head and shoulders. And be careful not to shoot your leg out into the extended position so that you jar your knee—*stretch* it out, feeling the muscles in the back of the thigh work.

EXERCISE 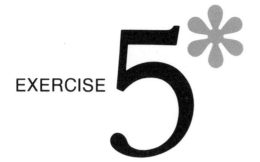 5 *

DOUBLE LEG STRETCH

Once you've stretched out each leg, this exercise can really work the muscles of the abdominal area and further limber your groin, hamstrings, and neck/shoulder area.

1 This time, bring both knees to the chest, each hand grasping an ankle, both feet flexed. As before, during the inhalation flex both knees as much as possible.

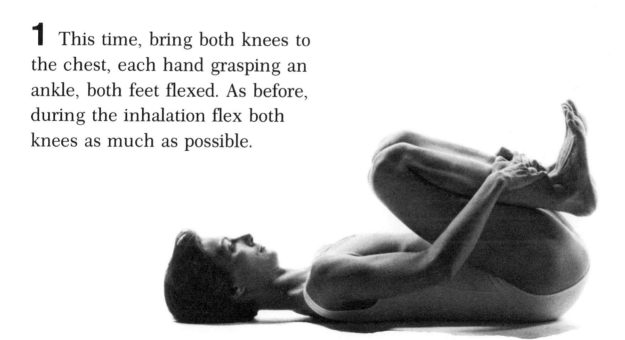

2 Exhale, contract the abdominal muscles, and raise the head, chin toward the chest; then extend both legs at about a 45-degree angle with the floor, arms parallel to your extended legs.

3 Inhale and draw your knees back to your chest.

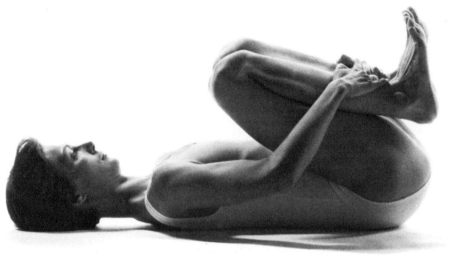

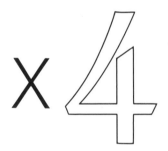 Do the exercise four times; then return to the relaxed base position.

In both this and the previous exercise, avoid any "crunching" or collapsing in the middle — keep your rib cage and spine long and stretched. Make sure you don't bring your legs so high that the tailbone, or coccyx, comes up off the floor, for then you won't be getting the benefits of the exercise. On the other hand, be careful that you don't let your legs extend too close to the floor, for this can put a little strain on your lower back. If you feel any twinges in your lower back when doing this exercise, raise your legs a bit. Keep all movements slow and even, with breath and action accompanying each other.

EXERCISE 6 *

SITTING ARM AND LEG STRETCH

Both this and the following exercise work the hamstrings, keeping the legs flexible and "stretched out." (Especially in men, this is an area that tends to get tight.) This series of movements is good preparation for any activity involving the legs — even walking.

1 Sit upright, with knees straight and feet flexed, causing your heels to be raised slightly from the floor. Keep your back straight.

2 Inhale, stretching the arms as far as you can toward the ceiling but keeping your shoulders down.

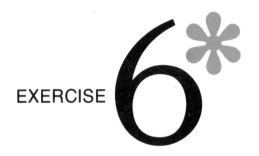

3 When you exhale, contract the abdominal muscles, reach even higher, and then, with a controlled sweeping motion, bring your head down, chin to your chest, bend over, and reach past the toes. Keep your arms beside your ears and parallel to the legs. It may help to imagine that you're actually reaching right across the ceiling and down the wall you're facing.

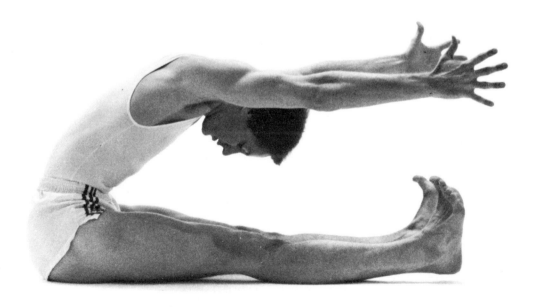

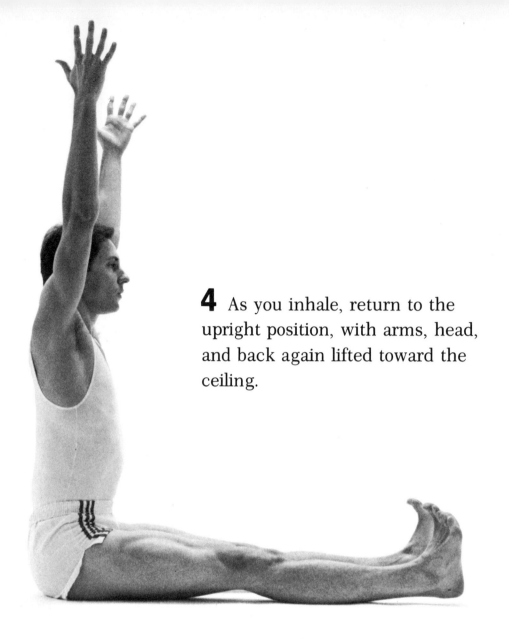

4 As you inhale, return to the upright position, with arms, head, and back again lifted toward the ceiling.

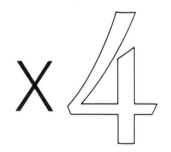

X4

After four stretches, on the fifth stretch proceed right into . . .

EXERCISE **7** ✱ **SITTING
LOWER BACK
STRETCH**

1 Continue bending forward,
reaching farther past the toes.
Feet remain flexed, heels slightly
raised. Now grasp your ankles
lightly.

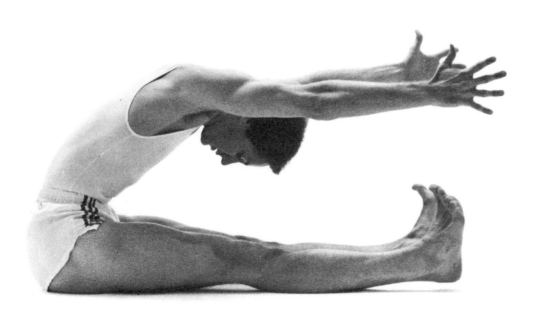

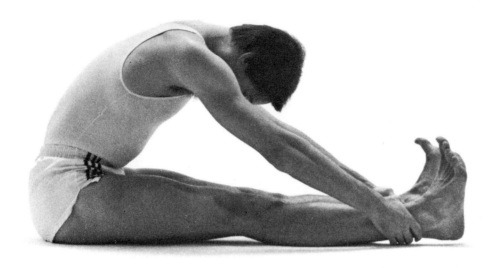

2 As you exhale with a contraction of the abdominal muscles, *slowly* bring your chest closer to your knees. On breathing in, relax the pull slightly and let the abdominal area fill with air. Each time you perform the stretching movement, apply a little more force than the time before.

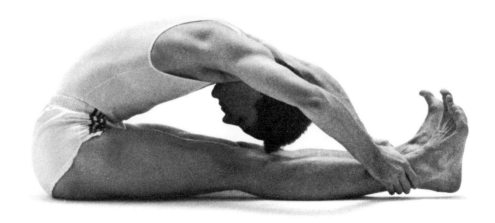

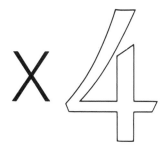 Perform the exercise four times.

In both this and the previous exercise, you should have the sensation that it's the contraction of the abdominal muscles that pulls you over — or lower, as the case may be. Pull the abdominals *in,* reach *out.* In EXER-CISE 7, the point is not to bend low, but to stretch out long. That's why you should aim to bring your *chest* — not your head — close to the knees. You get a longer stretch this way. *Special Note:* Frequently we mention the straight leg, and it *is* good to work with the leg as straight as possible. But by all means avoid locking the knees; stretching should be done with the knees relaxed, so there's no extreme pull in the lower back. Stretching with a locked knee can also overstretch the hamstrings, eventually causing problems in the cartilage. If you find your knees are locking, relax the flex in your foot and concentrate on keeping the backs of the thighs on the floor all the way down to the knee. This should help you achieve a relaxed stretch.

EXERCISE **8** ✽ SMALL BRIDGE

This is one of the most important exercises in the Nickolaus Technique, simple though it may seem. Doing it five times is enough to relax the lower back after the previous exercise. If you increase the number of repetitions, the movement will help to firm the buttocks, flatten the stomach, align the spine, and work the thigh and groin muscles. Overall, this exercise is a great "aligner" of the body.

1 Resume the initial breathing/relaxation position, arms at your sides, chin toward the chest, neck pressed down, lower back on the floor, shoulders relaxed, and feet turned slightly in.

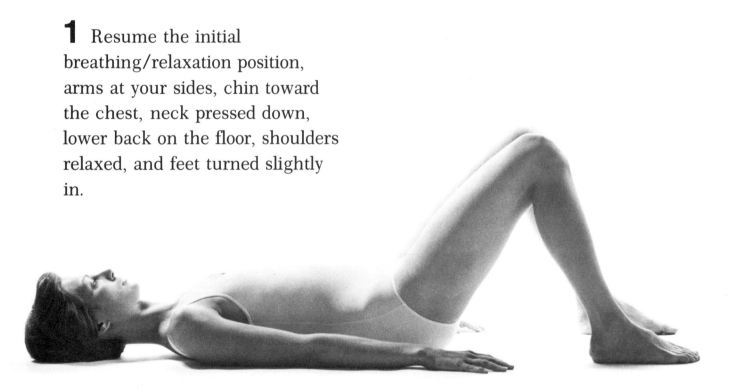

2 Inhale. . . . Then, breathing out, contract your lower abdominal muscles until the contraction pulls your tailbone under; at the same time, contract the buttocks muscles — much as if you were doing a slow "bump." Press your waist to the floor and apply slight resistance with your feet against the floor. Your tailbone should curl under, so that it comes slightly off the floor.

3 Now inhale, allowing your lower back to come back down to the floor.

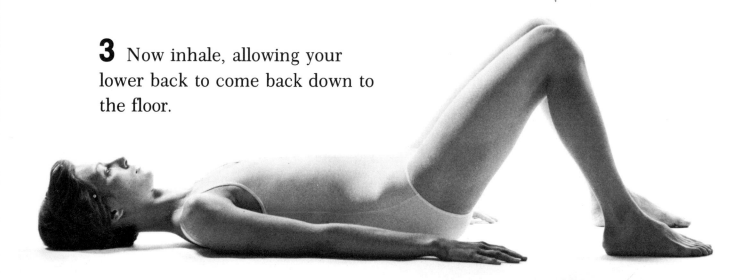

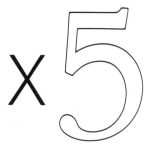

Do the exercise at least five times — more, if you want to increase the effect.

If you're doing this one right, you should feel a stretch in the upper thigh and groin, and a strong tightening of the buttocks. You should *not* feel any tension in the neck or shoulders.

Concentrate on the sensation and image of "rolling" up and down the spine, vertebra by vertebra, rather than pushing the pelvic area up in the air.

EXERCISE 9 THE "V"

This exercise stretches the inner thighs and strengthens the lower abdominal and seat muscles, greatly expanding the natural range of action in the lower body.

1 Lie down, back on the floor, hands at the sides, knees bent on the chest. Throughout this exercise, the lower back is kept on the floor, the feet are flexed, and the shoulders are relaxed.

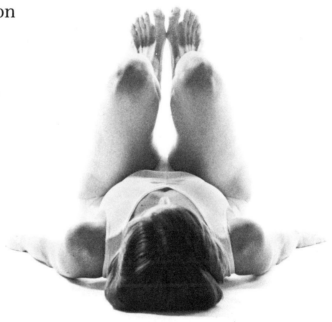

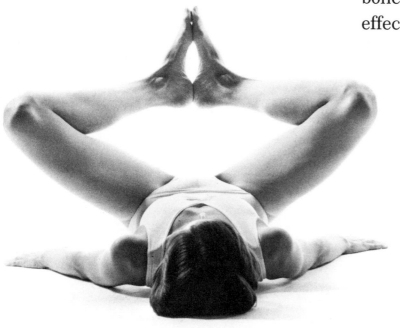

2 Inhale, and open the knees; bring the soles of your feet together, with toes, heels, and balls of the feet in contact with each other. Your heels should be brought as close to the pubic bone as flexibility allows. The effect is a sort of "frog-leg" look.

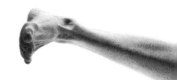

3 Exhale, contract the abdominal muscles, and—reaching through the heels—stretch the legs out in a V position. Extend the legs as far as possible while still keeping them at a right angle to the torso.

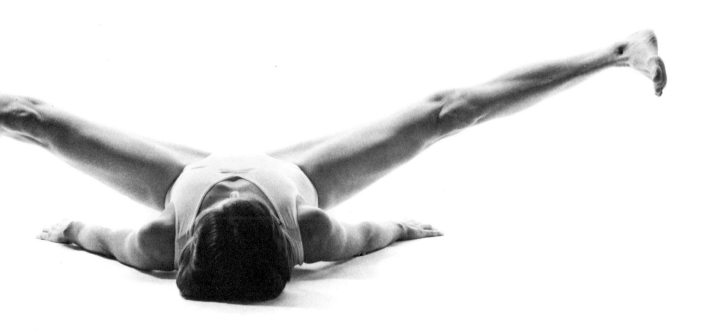

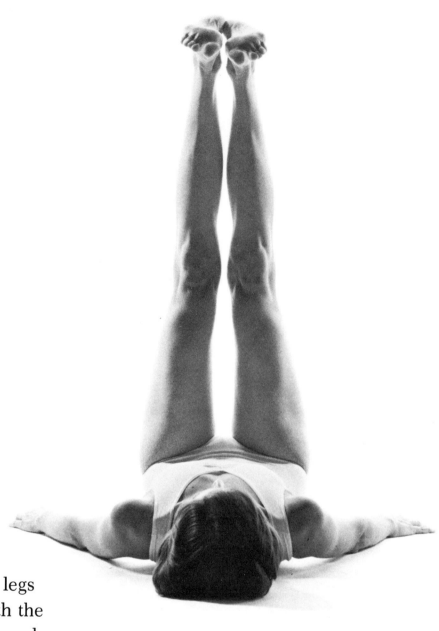

4 Inhale as you bring the legs
slowly up and together, with the
knees straight. Keep feet flexed.

5 Exhale, contracting the abdomen and using the contraction to draw the knees back toward your chest.

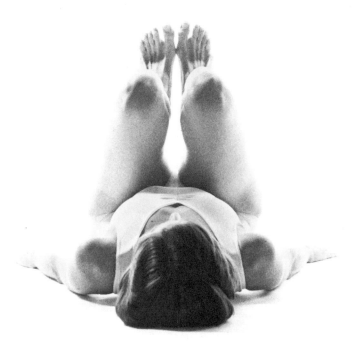

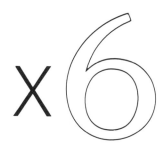 Perform the entire sequence six times.

If you feel any sensation in your lower back while doing this exercise, you are not doing it properly. Make sure your entire back, especially the area back of your waist, is pressed flat against the floor. When doing Step 4, be careful not to let your legs tilt away from you toward the floor, because this will put the strain on your back, instead of on your thighs and abdomen.

EXERCISE 10 SPINAL STRETCH

This is a wonderful exercise that releases any pressure on your spine, exactly as if you were hanging by your hands from a bar. In the case of rigid spines, it gently separates the vertebrae and releases compression of the disks, providing a kind of spinal traction. It also works on the lateral muscles of the arms to keep them toned and firm.

1 Still lying on the floor, bend your knees; your feet should be slightly turned in, your arms resting on the floor over your head. Inhale.

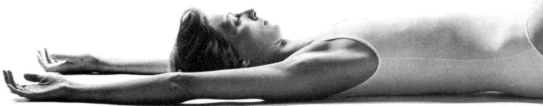

2 As you exhale, contract the lower abdominal muscles, gently push your spine against the floor, contract your buttocks, and bring your rib cage down to push the air out of your lungs. Reach for the wall behind you. *Really* reach.

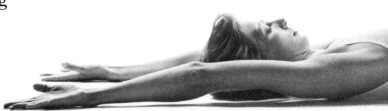

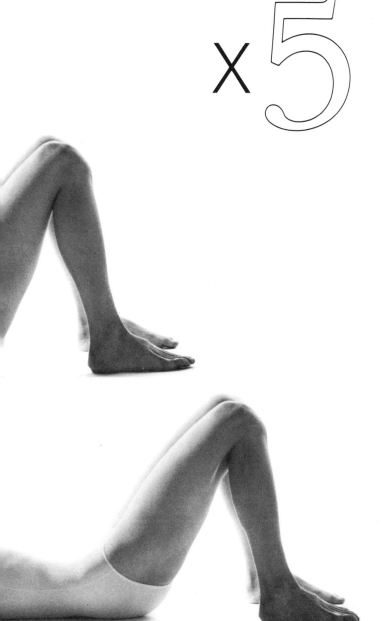

X5 Do the exercise five times.

You should feel a long, even stretch on exhalation, almost as if there were ropes around your wrists, pulling you as in traction. If you feel any tightness or tension in your back or shoulders, stop. Relax. Now start again, concentrating on exhaling a long, even column of breath and dropping your shoulder blades as you reach.

This exercise places the spine in the correct position for upper body carriage. Learn the feeling and hold on to it; you should strive for the same sensation when you are standing, sitting, and walking.

11

SHOULDER STRETCH

This stretch makes the shoulder area loose and flexible, works the pectoral muscle, and stimulates circulation in your upper body. An advantage of this simple exercise is that it can also be done sitting up, at your desk, during a break in housework, or whenever.

1 Lie on your back, knees bent, as in previous exercise, and place your hands on your chest.

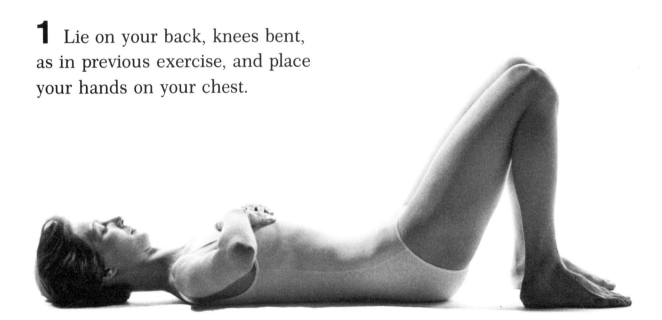

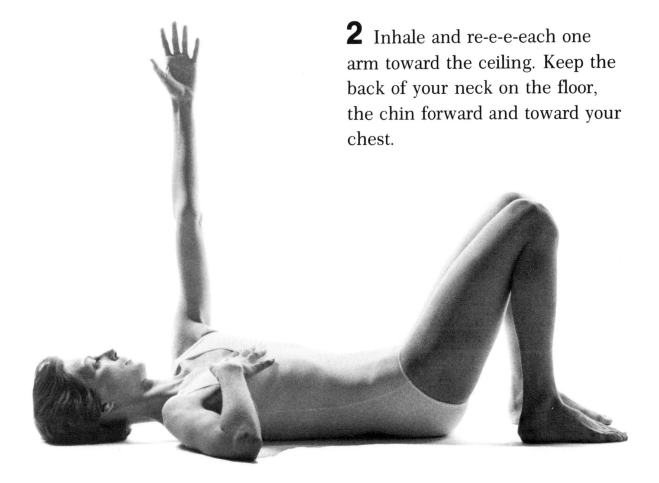

2 Inhale and re-e-e-each one arm toward the ceiling. Keep the back of your neck on the floor, the chin forward and toward your chest.

3 Exhale, replacing the hand gently on the chest. Repeat with the other arm, then with both together.

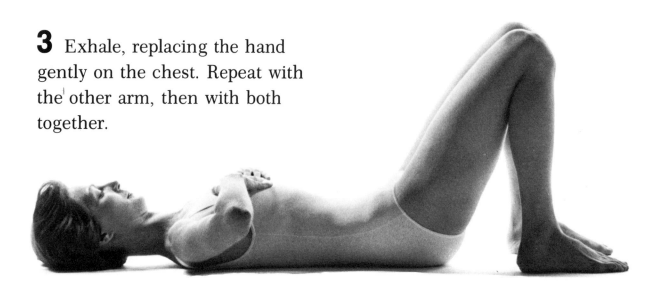

X 4 Perform the sequence four times.

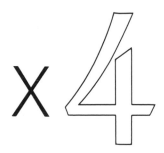

This is the one Nickolaus exercise where you inhale instead of exhale on the effort. In the Shoulder Stretch, the inhalation combined with the reach upward makes the muscle on the inside of your arm really work and stretches the pectoral and shoulder girdle. Your shoulder, arm, hand, and chest should all tingle afterward; if they don't, breathe deeper, reach harder.

EXERCISE **12** NECK AND UPPER BACK STRETCH

Tension in the shoulder area often leads to headaches; this exercise releases tension there. It also gives you greater freedom of movement in your upper body.

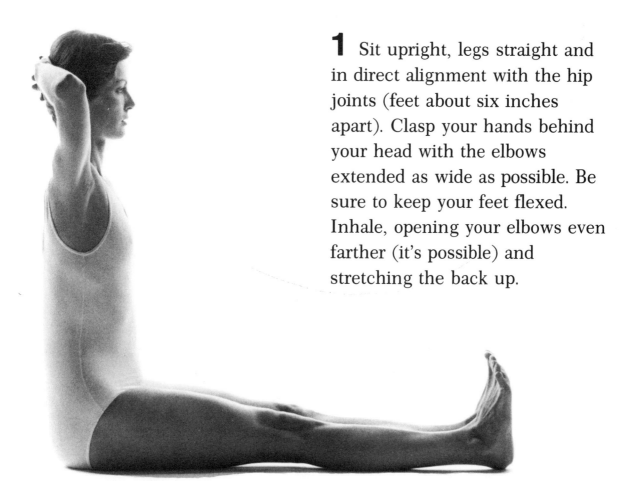

1 Sit upright, legs straight and in direct alignment with the hip joints (feet about six inches apart). Clasp your hands behind your head with the elbows extended as wide as possible. Be sure to keep your feet flexed. Inhale, opening your elbows even farther (it's possible) and stretching the back up.

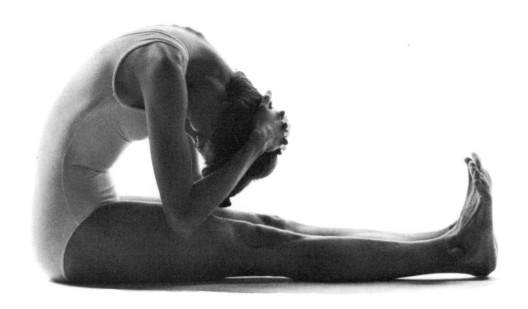

2 As you exhale, contract your abdominal muscles, lower your head, let your elbows come closer together, pull your chin to your chest, and round your lower back. Do not press your head down with your hands. Try to touch your chin to your chest and let the abdominal contraction pull you into a curled position. You will feel a real stretch — sometimes almost a painful one — first in your neck, then across the shoulders, then (a little bit) in your middle back.

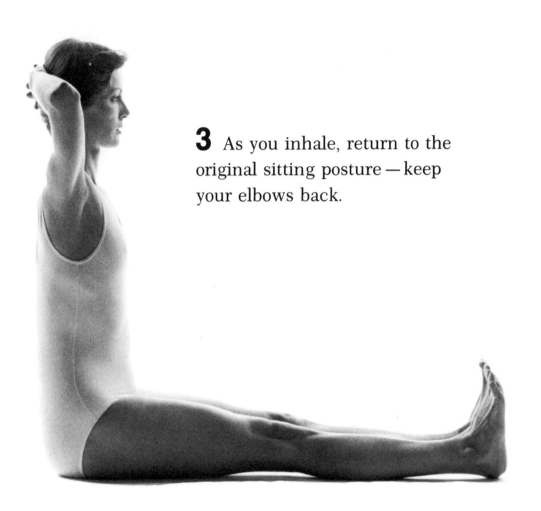

3 As you inhale, return to the original sitting posture — keep your elbows back.

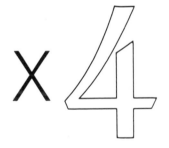

Perform the movement four times; then, on the fifth time, hold the downward position for . . .

EXERCISE **13** MIDDLE BACK
STRETCH

This movement intensifies the effect of the
last exercise, reaching the stretch farther
down, into the middle and lower back area.
The movement is good for the most common
form of lower back pain, discomfort from poor
posture.

1 Inhale in the downward
position of the last exercise, but
do not sit up; then exhale so that
your stomach feels as if it will
touch your backbone, and move
the top of the head farther toward
the thighs. Try to touch your
navel with your nose (you can't
really do it, but *try*). Don't
bounce; use consistent, gentle
stretching pressure.

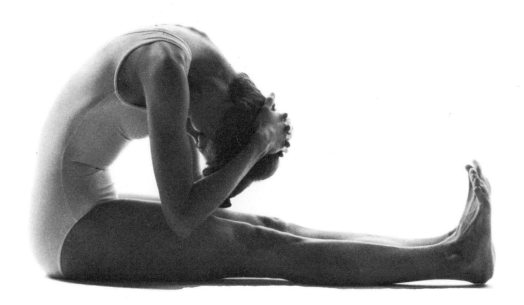

2 Hold the position; inhale and release the pull; exhale, repeating the stretch. On breathing in, just let the abdominals relax; when you breathe out, do so with a strong abdominal contraction.

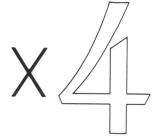

Do the stretch four times.

In both this and the previous exercise, you should feel a real pulling in of your abdominal area when you exhale, as if you were going to touch it to your spine. At first, it may be difficult to feel the stretch very far down the spine; but as you continue to do the exercise, you'll feel it more and more toward your middle and lower back.

EXERCISE **14** HEAD ROLLS

These are excellent for relieving tension headaches and stretching the sides of your neck, an area that tends to get tight and inflexible. You can do this exercise just about anywhere you're able to keep your back erect.

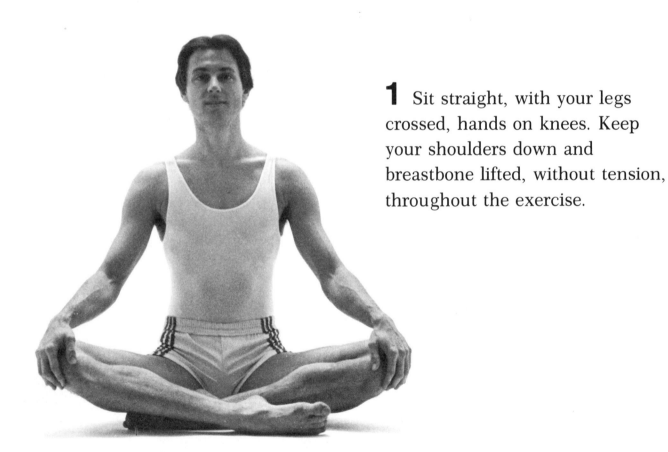

1 Sit straight, with your legs crossed, hands on knees. Keep your shoulders down and breastbone lifted, without tension, throughout the exercise.

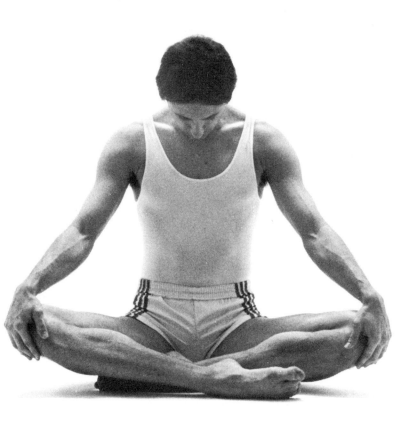

2 Breathing in, allow your chin to drop forward on your chest.

3 Roll the head to the left so your left ear is parallel to your left shoulder; then let your head roll to the back, stretching your chin toward the ceiling. Keep your shoulders down — do *not* let them shrug up to meet your head.

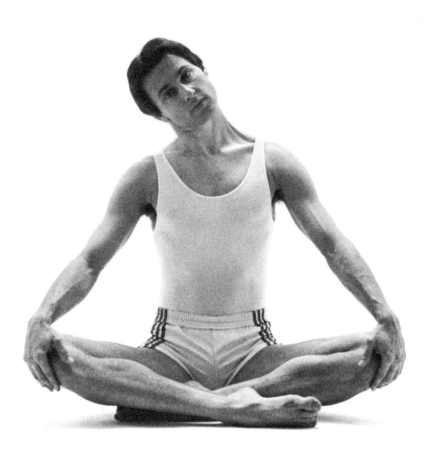

4 Continue the motion while
breathing out, as you roll your
head around to the right shoulder
and then roll it forward so your
chin rests on your chest.

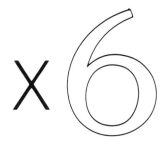 Do the rolls six times to the left, six times to the right.

If you are normally tense, spend a lot of time sitting at a desk, or are prone to tension headaches, your neck is probably very inflexible, and this exercise may seem very painful at first. Do it slowly and resist the impulse to let the muscles contract at the first twinge of a stretch. Relax. Press your shoulders down and keep rolling your head around slowly. When you can finally do this smoothly you will find it relieves tension you may not even have realized was there.

EXERCISE **15** ROLL-UPS

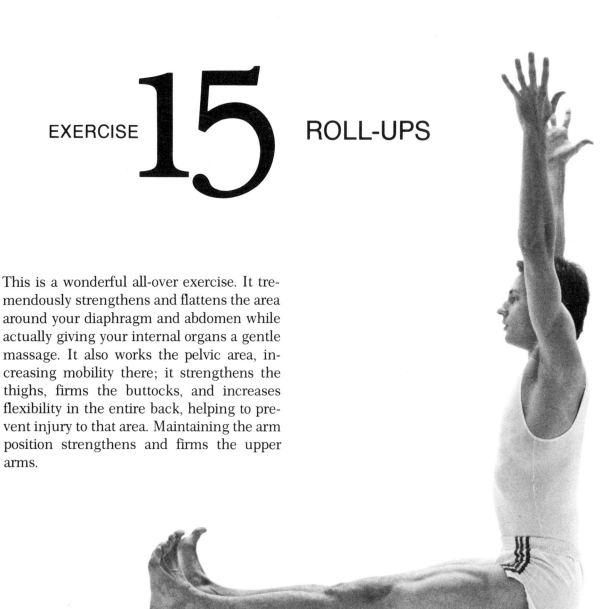

This is a wonderful all-over exercise. It tremendously strengthens and flattens the area around your diaphragm and abdomen while actually giving your internal organs a gentle massage. It also works the pelvic area, increasing mobility there; it strengthens the thighs, firms the buttocks, and increases flexibility in the entire back, helping to prevent injury to that area. Maintaining the arm position strengthens and firms the upper arms.

1 Sit with your legs straight, feet flexed, and arms beside the ears, reaching for the ceiling, and stretch up, as if trying to touch the ceiling with your fingertips. Breathe in.

2 Then, as you breathe out, contract your abdominal muscles and tuck the pelvis so that you slowly roll back, one vertebra at a time. Keep your back *round*.

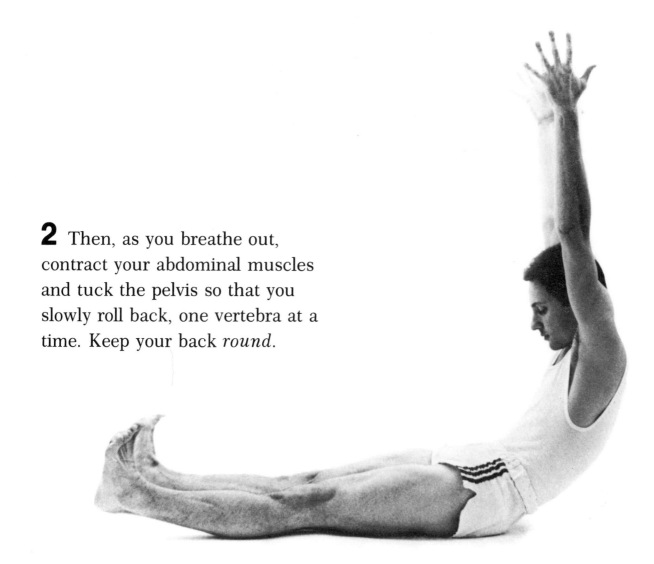

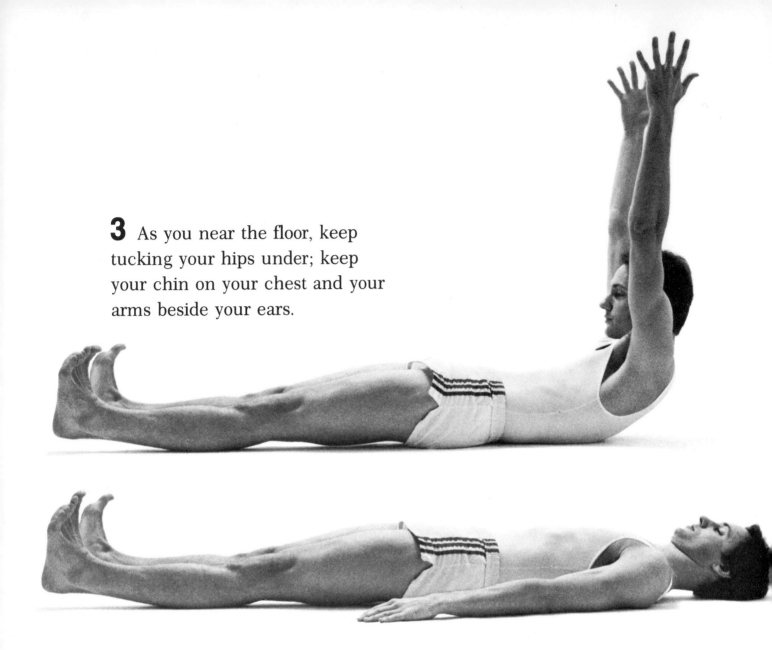

3 As you near the floor, keep tucking your hips under; keep your chin on your chest and your arms beside your ears.

4 After your shoulders touch the floor, place your arms by your sides, rest your head on the floor and relax briefly.

5 As you breathe in again, lift
your head and place your chin on
your chest; raise your arms
straight up toward the ceiling,
again keeping them beside your
ears.

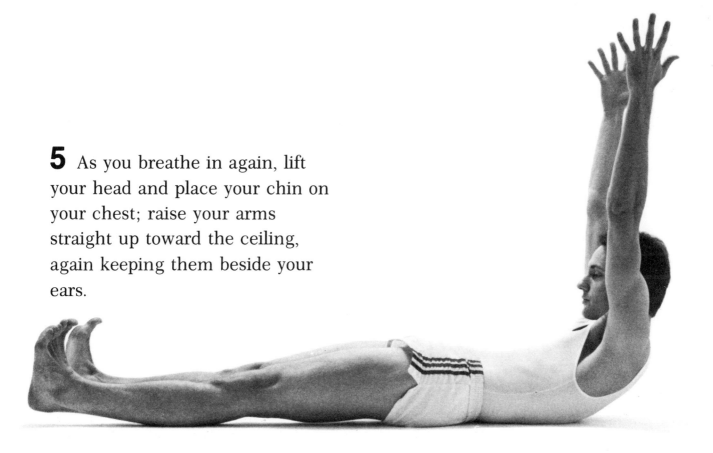

6 Exhaling, press the lower abdominal muscles toward the spine and slowly roll up with the back rounded — again, one vertebra at a time — to the original sitting position. (If you run out of breath at any point, stop the motion, inhale, and while breathing out, continue the motion.)

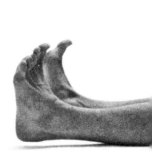

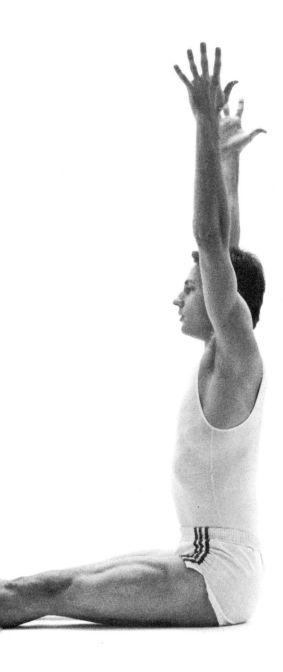

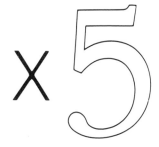

Do this exercise five times.

This exercise is not easy; without practice, only a few people can roll up from the floor at all, let alone do it correctly. In the beginning, you can bend your knees slightly and place your hands on your thighs to help yourself up, until you acquire the necessary strength in the abdomen and flexibility in the lower back to do the exercise as described above. Placing your hands on your thighs will, in fact, insure that you round the back as you come up, instead of letting it straighten out, which would put strain on your back muscles and might cause you to build up bulging stomach muscles instead of the flat ones you want. As you get stronger and can take your hands off your thighs, make a conscious effort as you roll up to *contract* yourself into a rolled-up position and not to push yourself up with a straight back.

EXERCISE 16 THE BIRD

This is an old yoga exercise that strengthens the lower back muscles and tightens the buttocks and the muscles in the back of the legs. The pace is slow, and the lifts are slight.

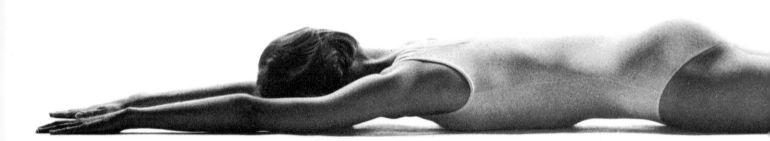

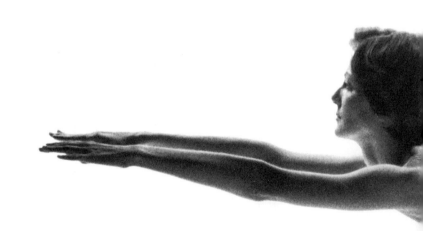

1 Lie on your stomach with your arms outstretched above your head.

2 As you exhale, contract the abdominal muscles and buttocks, and lift the arms, head, and legs slightly off the floor.

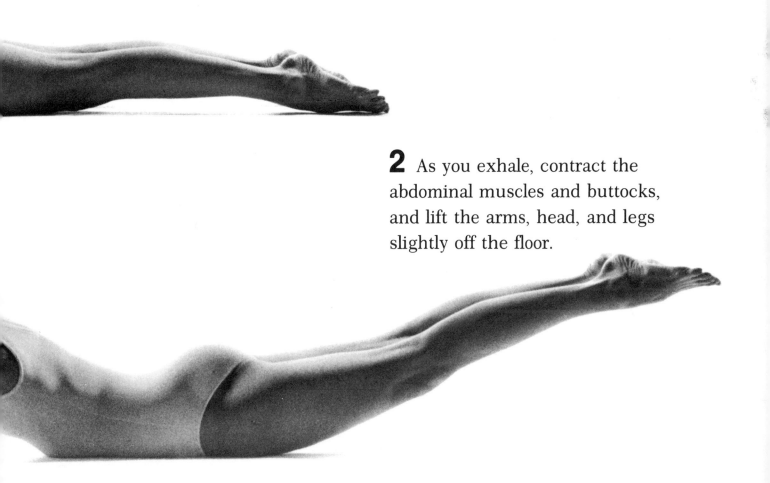

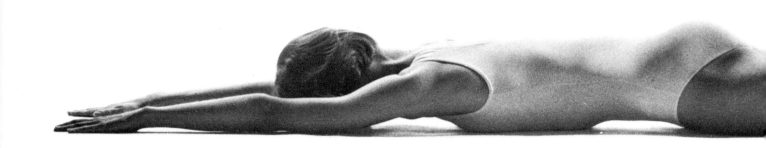

3 As you inhale, slowly lower
arms, head and legs.

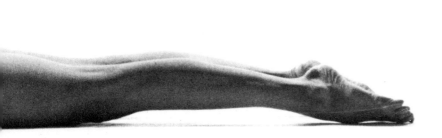

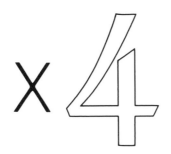 × 4   Do the exercise four times, slightly increasing the lift each time.

You should feel this exercise in your buttocks, your abdomen, and the backs of your thighs. A slight burning sensation in the buttocks or the backs of the thighs, in fact, means you're *really* working. You should not, however, feel any twinges in your lower back. If you do, you are not concentrating hard enough on the abdomen and buttocks. Really work on these, and you should relieve all strain on the back.

EXERCISE **17** REST

Here is an exercise that doesn't make you work. It just relaxes you and gives the back a gentle stretch, helping you to recover from the previous exercises and prepare for the ones that follow.

1 Kneel; then curl up in a fetal position so that your chest rests on your thighs and your buttocks touch your heels, or get as close to that position as you can. Your feet are extended and the tops of your toes are on the floor. Your back should be rounded, your head tucked under so the *top* of the head, not the forehead, is resting on the floor. Your arms are relaxed at the sides of the body, with fingers resting near the toes.

2 Hold the position for about a minute, breathing deeply.

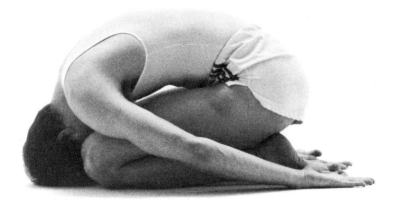

There are two rest periods in the program, and each occurs after an exertion in the lower back. Don't skip them. If you have any doubts about how much of an exercise the rest is, "listen" to your lower back muscles as you inhale deeply. Feel them stretch?

EXERCISE 18 LEG LIFTS

Leg lifts are not easy — in fact, students often groan when they reach this point in class. But the lifts are a key part of the Technique. They strengthen, tone, and firm the thigh muscles; and they normalize them, slimming a heavy thigh and contouring a skinny one. In addition, the exercise strengthens the lower abdominals and virtually the entire back. This strengthening of the upper body, as well as the thigh work, will transfer to the later exercises for posture and alignment — and eventually, to the movements of your everyday life.

1 Sit erect, with your knees straight and feet flexed, about hip-width apart. Place the back of one hand against the lower back; place the back of your other hand against the palm of your first hand. Throughout this exercise, *hold your back straight.* Otherwise, you'll work only the muscles in the top thigh, making them bunch up instead of growing long and supple. Keep your shoulders relaxed and your chin *somewhat* lowered, maintaining the back of the neck and head in straight alignment with the spine.

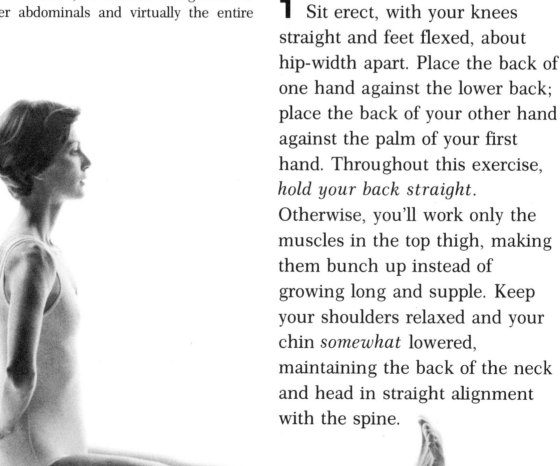

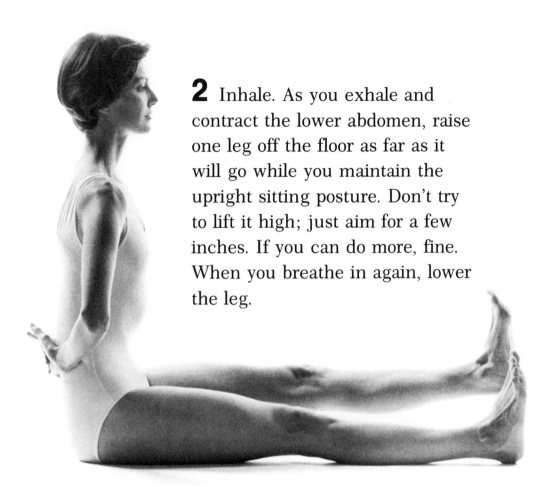

2 Inhale. As you exhale and contract the lower abdomen, raise one leg off the floor as far as it will go while you maintain the upright sitting posture. Don't try to lift it high; just aim for a few inches. If you can do more, fine. When you breathe in again, lower the leg.

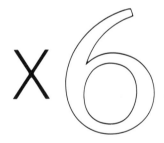

This is a toughie, so take it easy at first; do it only six times with each leg. Then try to work up to twenty times with each leg.

In a sense, these leg lifts should be the same kind of experience as running a mile: You should feel you're fully using your body—in this case really fighting to sit up and out of your hips. The exercise is quite severe and requires sustained effort—especially if you're anxious to reduce the size of your thighs. Only continuous movement will "overwork" the muscle so that it becomes smaller and tighter. Remember, the point of the exercise is not how high you can lift your leg—it should never be more than six inches off the floor—but how straight you can keep your back.

EXERCISE **19** ## SIDE LEG LIFTS

Side leg lifts are wonderful for eliminating those fleshy deposits on the sides of the legs, just below the buttocks. They also work the abdominals and generally strengthen the legs.

1 Lie on one side. The bottom leg should be outstretched straight, in the same line as the torso; if this is too difficult at first, it's okay to bend the bottom leg until the movement gets easier. The top leg is straight in front—ideally, perpendicular to the torso, though again it may take some time to work up to this. Hold your top leg and knee straight, with your foot flexed, throughout these movements. The head is supported with the right hand if you're lifting the left leg, and vice versa. Bend your other arm at the elbow, and rest the hand on the floor in front of the chest at a right angle to your body. (It sounds more complicated than it is—take a look at the picture.) The top shoulder should be slightly forward and the back gently rounded; the top hip must be directly above the bottom hip, so you're lying in the correct alignment.

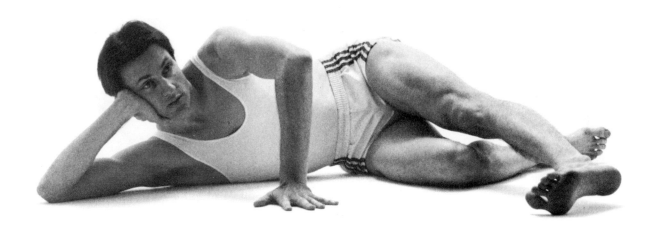

2 As you breathe out, pull your lower abdominal muscles to the back, tighten *both* buttocks, and raise your top leg about two feet off the ground. Use your buttocks muscles to make sure you don't displace the top leg when you lift it. When you breathe in, lower the leg slowly. The heel of the lifted leg should be slightly higher than its big toe.

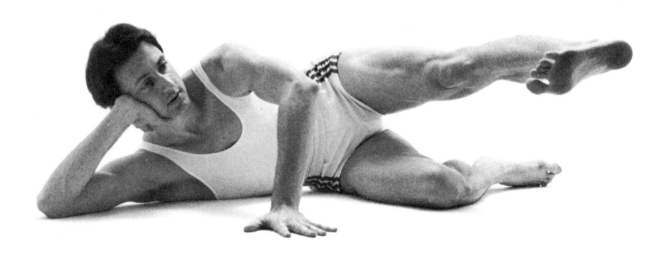

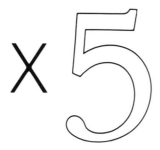

×5   Again, start with five lifts and work up to twenty on each side.

Many conventional exercise programs incorporate a movement that involves lifting the leg sideways and is supposed to slim the muscles at the side of the thigh and under the buttock. Unfortunately, these exercises rarely do more than give the hip joint a workout, since no one ever tells you to keep the hips completely stationary, one above the other. If you allow the top hip to displace as you raise your leg, you are letting the hip joint take the strain that should be assumed by the muscles surrounding the joint. If you feel any sensation along your sides, that means you're letting your hip come up; concentrate harder on contracting your abdomen, clenching your buttocks, and reaching out with your heel. Lift the leg straight up from the floor, not on the diagonal, and keep it in the same plane during the lift; don't let it flop or wave around. You should feel a burning sensation in the buttocks, or down the backs of the thighs, when doing this properly.

EXERCISE 20 THE BOW

After all the work your thigh muscles get in the leg lifts, they need a simple stretch. This exercise elongates the front of the thigh, and helps your body to recover from the leg lifts. The exercise will further limber your lower back.

1 Lie on your stomach, with your legs bent, your hands stretched back to grasp your ankles.

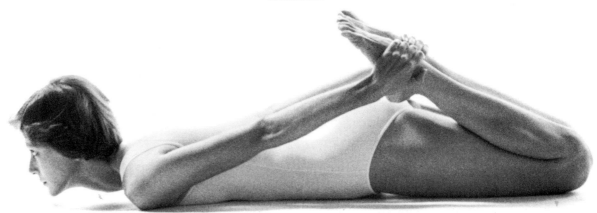

2 When you breathe out,
contract the buttock muscles,
push the lower abdominal
muscles to the spine, and lift
your chest and knees off the
floor. Keep your knees together
and your feet lifted toward the
ceiling. When you reach the top
of your stretch, tilt your chin
back to stretch your neck and get
a good pull on your stomach
muscles.

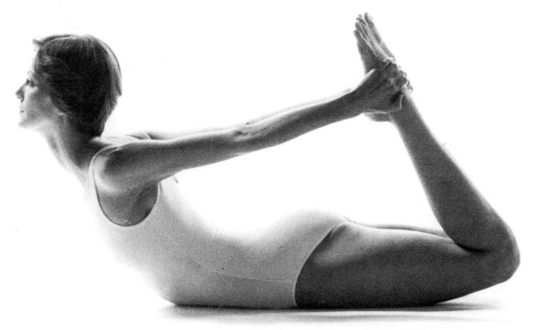

3 As you inhale, return to the initial position.

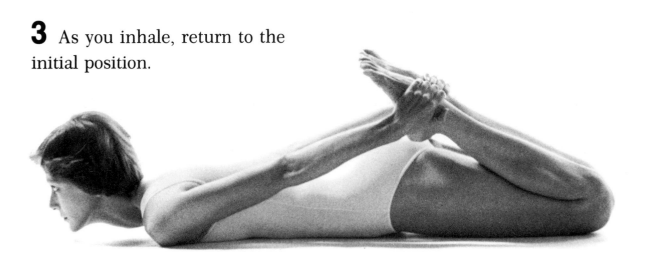

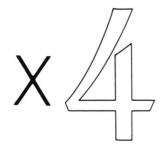

Do the exercise four times.

It's important to keep your knees together and to use your abdomen and buttocks to lift yourself up. If you feel any strain in your knees — which you don't want — make sure you're pressing them and your feet together as you rise. And if you feel any twinges in your back, work harder on contracting your abdomen.

EXERCISE **21** REST

1 Kneel; then assume the REST position, with back rounded and arms relaxed (for description and comments, see EXERCISE 17 on page 98).

2 Hold the position about a minute. Breathe.

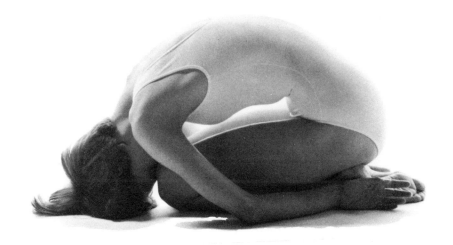

EXERCISE 22

SINGLE THIGH STRETCH

This exercise helps align the body and straighten the spine. It stretches out the front thigh muscles and those in the groin area and tones the buttocks and the back of the thigh.

1 Kneel on one knee and place the other foot in front for balance, with the weight slightly forward. (See picture for correct alignment — the forward leg forms a right angle.) Clasp your hands on your raised knee.

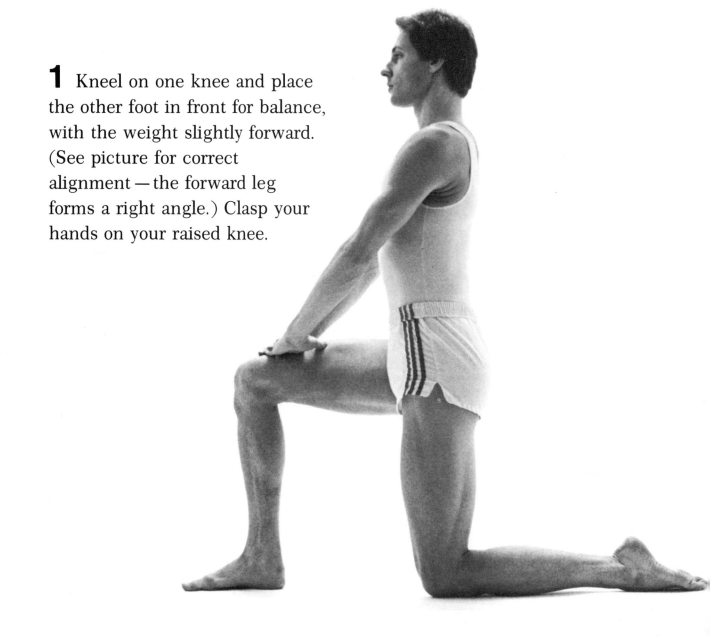

2 As you exhale, contract the lower abdominals, rotate the pelvis under, and pull down the lower back, tightening the buttocks — another mini-"bump." Your chest should be lifted and your shoulders down, free from tension.

3 As you inhale, relax and return to the initial position.

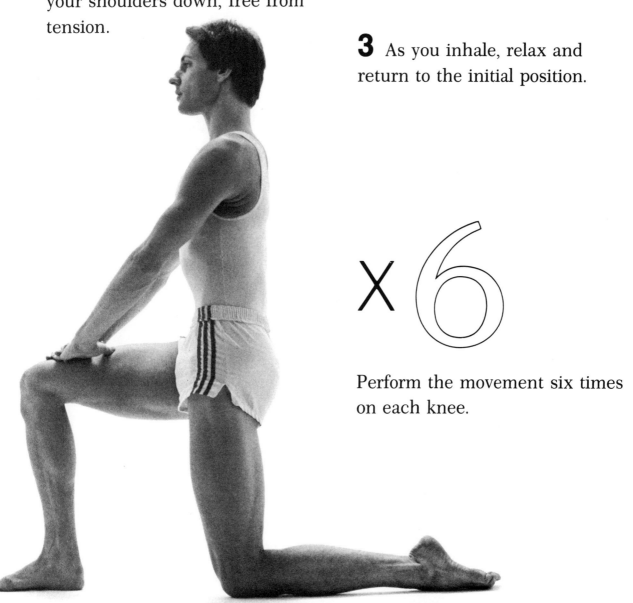

X 6

Perform the movement six times on each knee.

Avoid tension in the shoulders, bending or "collapsing" in the back. You should feel a pull along the sides of the thigh of the leg you're kneeling on.

23

DOUBLE THIGH STRETCH

This strengthens the muscles around your knee joint, crucial to avoiding injuries of the knee. The exercise also strengthens and stretches the front of your thigh. It's hard, in this exercise, to keep your body in the proper alignment; the effort to do so will make your entire torso stronger.

1 Kneel on both knees, arms held straight in front of your body, parallel to the floor. Keep your back straight. As you exhale, contract the lower abdominal muscles, tip your pelvis under, and tighten your buttock muscles.

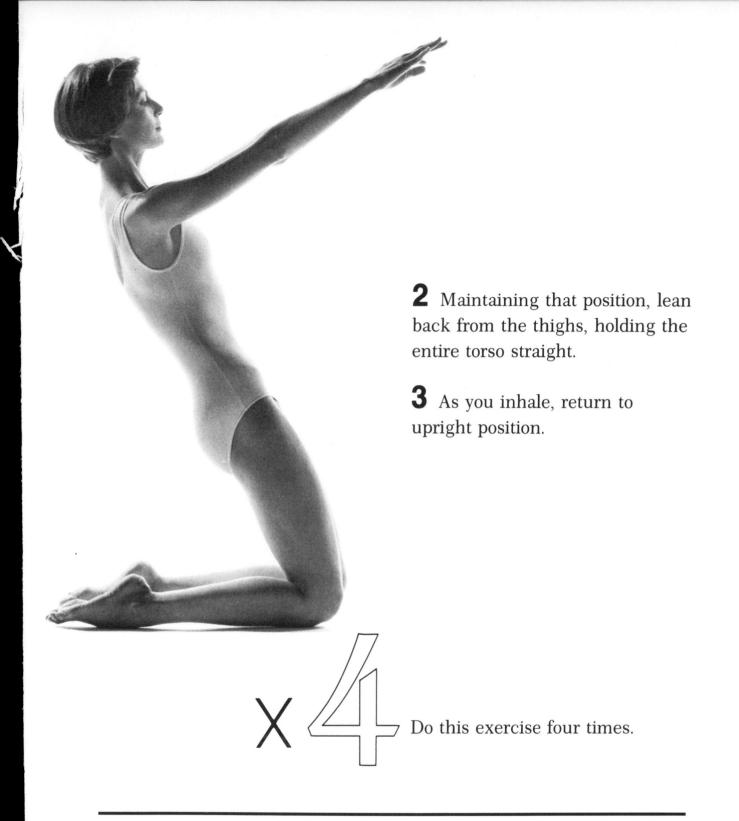

2 Maintaining that position, lean back from the thighs, holding the entire torso straight.

3 As you inhale, return to upright position.

X4 Do this exercise four times.

It's not as important to lean far back — a slight departure from the vertical is enough — as it is to keep the torso in a straight line. You should feel the muscles in the backs of your thighs and your buttocks working, and there shouldn't be any feeling of strain on your knees. If there is, try stretching your torso *long*, making your body *light* — so it doesn't put strain on the knee joint.

EXERCISE **24** INNER THIGH STRETCH WITH SPINAL ROTATION

This exercise stretches the inner thighs and hamstrings, areas important for physical activity — sports or just plain old housework. The more vigorous forms of activity can easily injure your inner thigh, and this exercise will help prevent such injury. The turning motion increases your spinal mobility.

1 Sit with your legs spread open in as wide a V as you can make, your feet flexed, knees straight, and arms raised over your head.

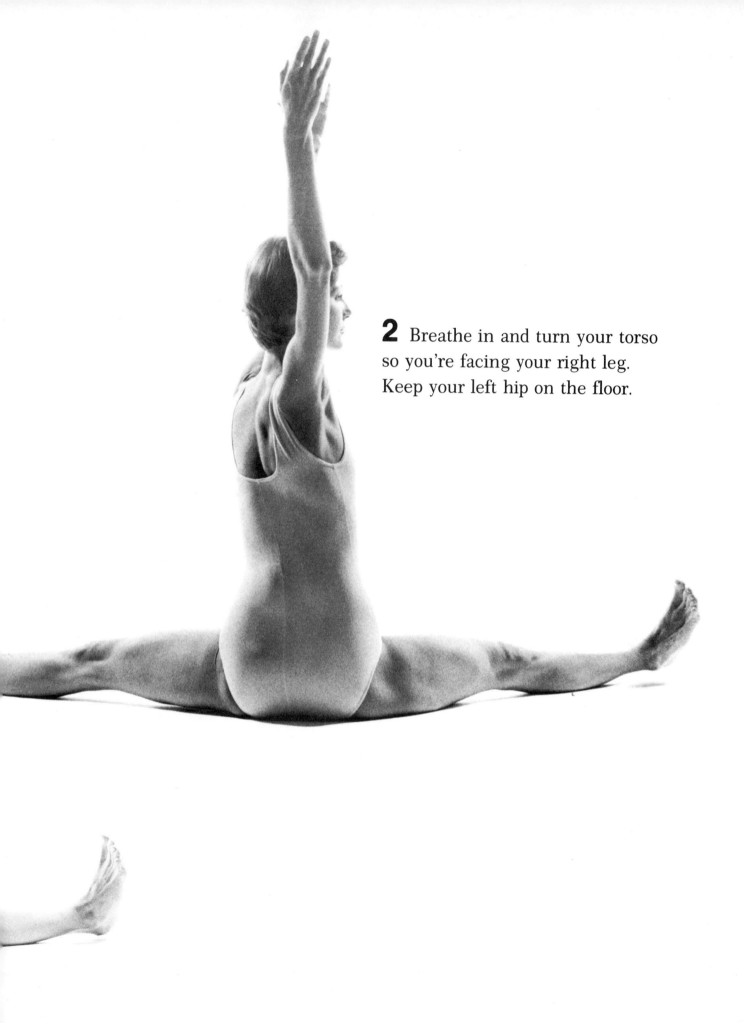

2 Breathe in and turn your torso
so you're facing your right leg.
Keep your left hip on the floor.

3 Breathe out, contract the lower abdominals and the buttocks, and lean over so that, if the movement were continued, both hands would reach past the right foot and the head would rest on the knee — don't worry if you're not actually able to stretch that far. Keep your left buttock on the floor during this stretch, and make sure both knees are *straight*, not bent, and your toes are pointing toward the ceiling.

4 Inhale and sit up. Turn to the left, exhale, and repeat the reaching movement.

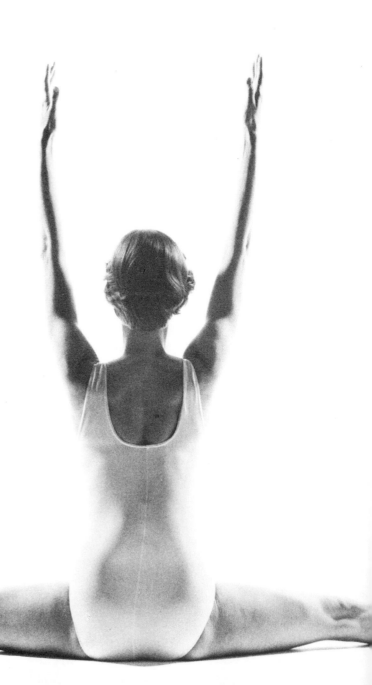

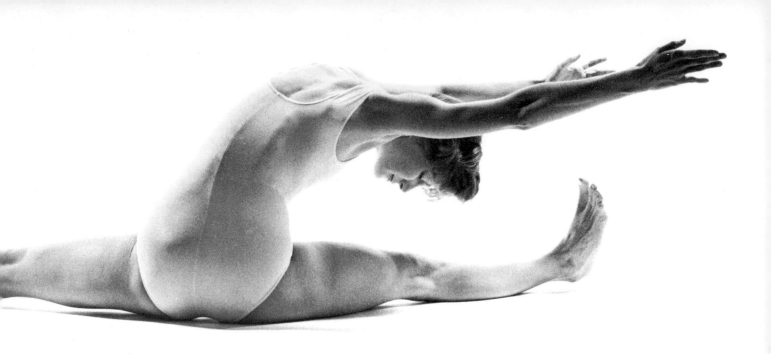

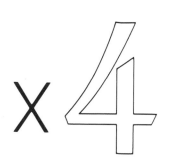 X 4 Stretch four times to each side.

Don't let the stretch toward your foot pull the opposite buttock off the floor. You should feel instead a very definite pull along the side opposite the direction you're reaching. That means you've placed your body properly and kept the placement.

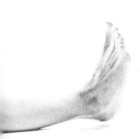

25

INNER THIGH AND LATERAL STRETCH

This exercise increases spinal mobility even further, and stretches the side muscles.

1 Stay in the same position as for the last exercise, but try to spread your legs somewhat wider — after the stretch of the previous exercise, you should be able to. Raise your arms above your head.

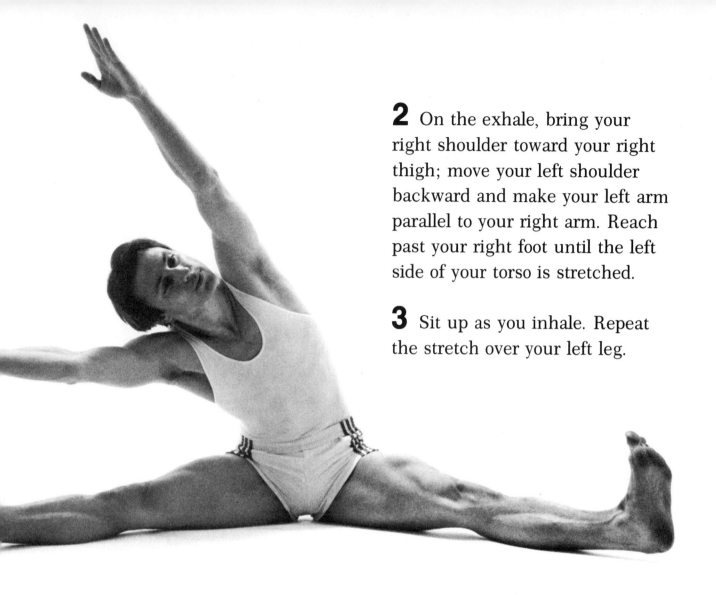

2 On the exhale, bring your right shoulder toward your right thigh; move your left shoulder backward and make your left arm parallel to your right arm. Reach past your right foot until the left side of your torso is stretched.

3 Sit up as you inhale. Repeat the stretch over your left leg.

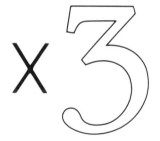

Do the exercise three times on each side.

Once again, keep both buttocks on the floor. The pull along the side opposite the direction you're reaching should be intensified with each repetition. Don't jerk or bounce; just maintain a slow, even pull in the direction of the stretch.

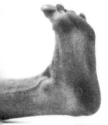

EXERCISE 26

TURNED-OUT LEG LIFT

Besides being good for the inner thighs, this exercise strengthens the muscles around the knee and is especially beneficial for a person with an injured knee.

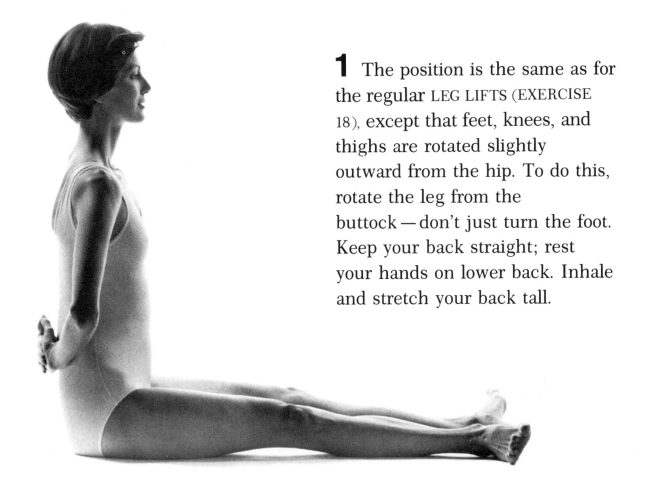

1 The position is the same as for the regular LEG LIFTS (EXERCISE 18), except that feet, knees, and thighs are rotated slightly outward from the hip. To do this, rotate the leg from the buttock — don't just turn the foot. Keep your back straight; rest your hands on lower back. Inhale and stretch your back tall.

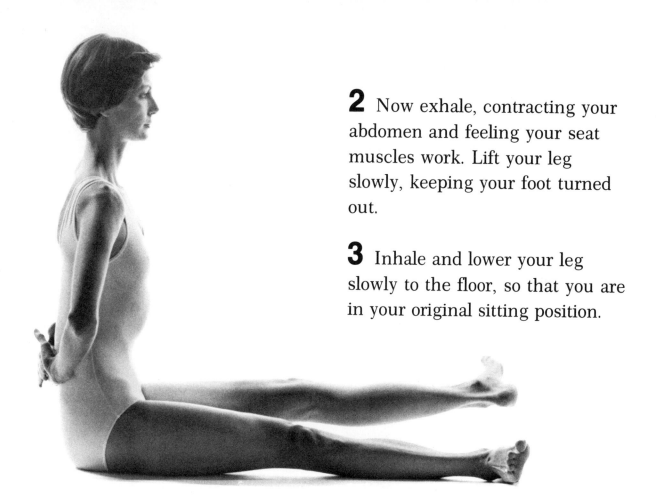

2 Now exhale, contracting your abdomen and feeling your seat muscles work. Lift your leg slowly, keeping your foot turned out.

3 Inhale and lower your leg slowly to the floor, so that you are in your original sitting position.

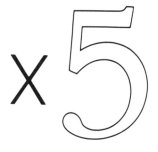

Do this exercise five times on each leg.

If you think of raising the heel on the lifts (no more than six inches), that should help you achieve the proper rotation. Again, don't worry if you can do the movement only a few times; as you grow stronger, you'll be able to do more.

EXERCISE **27**   THE SQUEEZE

This deceptively simple exercise tightens the buttocks and inner thighs and strengthens the pectoral muscles. It is a variation on EXERCISE 10, the SPINAL STRETCH. You strive for the same perfect alignment of the spine—this time, on your feet. It will improve your posture no end.

1 Stand with your weight on the balls of your feet. Keep your palms together, with fingers pointing upward, about six inches in front of your chest. Hold your fingertips level with your shoulders and your elbows up; arms and chest form a rectangle.

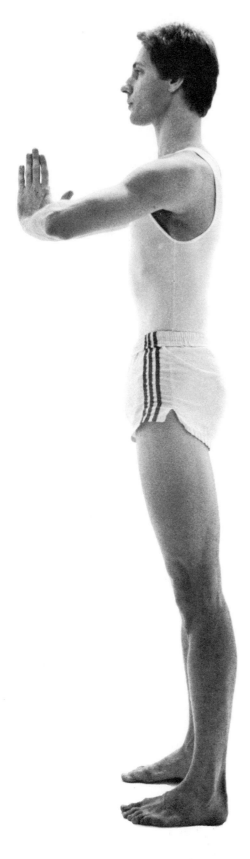

2 As you exhale, tuck your pelvis under, tighten your buttocks, and press your hands together. The back and knees are kept straight.

3 As you inhale, allow your hips to tip back slightly, and relax. Exhale and repeat.

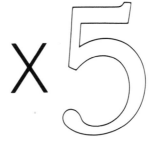

Do this five times.

When you tuck and exhale in this exercise, be careful not to lock your knees and rock outward on the outsides of your feet. Stand lightly and squarely on your feet, and think tall — stretch your spine upward as you tuck.

EXERCISE **28** STANDING LATERAL STRETCH

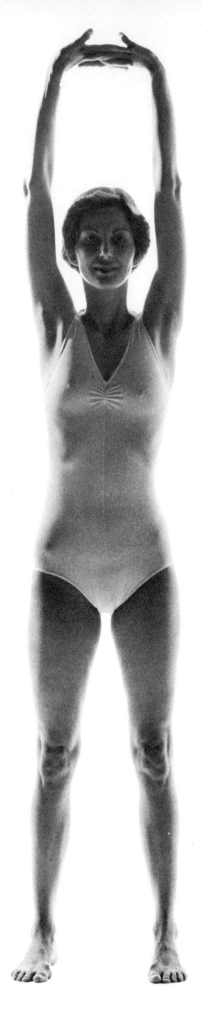

This is a good stretch to do after any kind of hard exercise. It tightens the buttocks and stretches the sides of the torso. Most people find this movement especially invigorating.

1 Stand straight, with legs apart, hands over your head, fingers intertwined, palms up.

2 As you exhale, contract the abdominal muscles, tuck your pelvis under and up, and lean to one side, keeping your weight evenly distributed on both feet. Your elbows should be completely extended, arms beside your ears.

3 Inhaling, return to original position. Repeat on the other side.

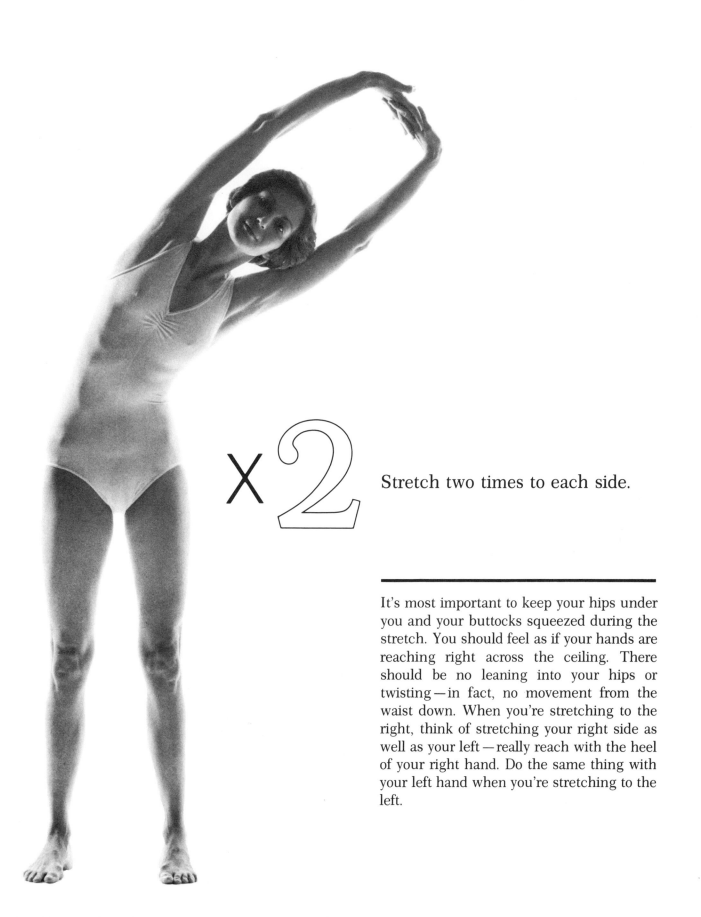

x2

Stretch two times to each side.

It's most important to keep your hips under you and your buttocks squeezed during the stretch. You should feel as if your hands are reaching right across the ceiling. There should be no leaning into your hips or twisting—in fact, no movement from the waist down. When you're stretching to the right, think of stretching your right side as well as your left—really reach with the heel of your right hand. Do the same thing with your left hand when you're stretching to the left.

EXERCISE **29** STANDING LEG AND BACK STRETCH

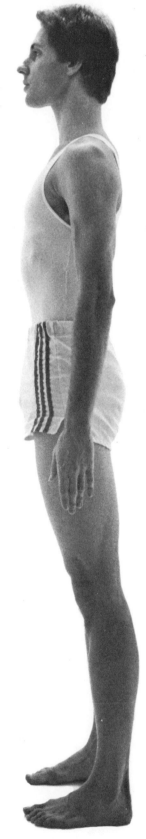

This exercise is excellent for circulation and makes a good pick-me-up if you've had a long day at a desk or in a plane or train or car. It and the SITTING LOWER BACK STRETCH (EXERCISE 7) provide the biggest stretch for the hamstrings.

1 Stand straight, your legs slightly apart and your weight on the balls of your feet.

2 Inhale. Imagine that your head is *very* heavy. Let your chin fall forward on your chest.

3 Exhale. Now let the weight of your head cause your shoulders to collapse forward very slowly. The weight of your entire upper body causes you to bend over *slowly* at the waist, with your arms hanging down like dead weight. The only thing that is keeping you from collapsing entirely is the contraction in your abdomen and buttocks muscles.

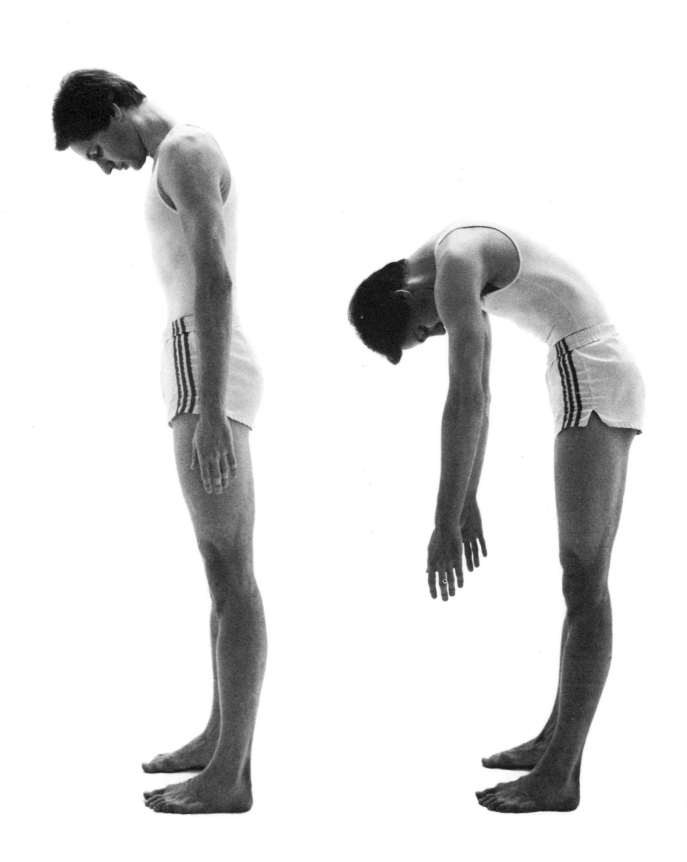

4 Grasp your ankles — or, if you can't reach your ankles, the backs of your calves.

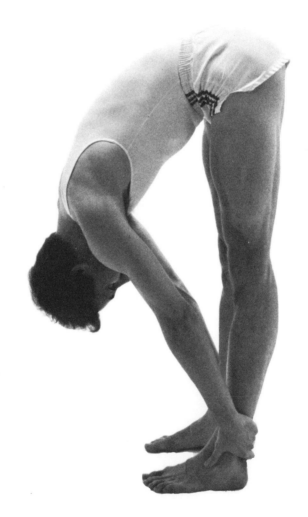

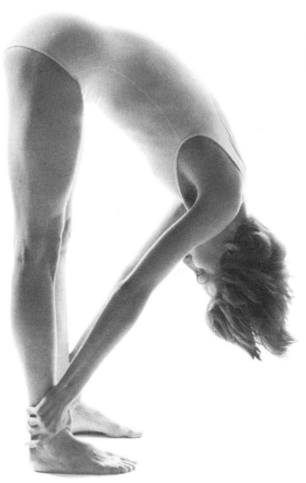

5 Now, staying in the same position, inhale.

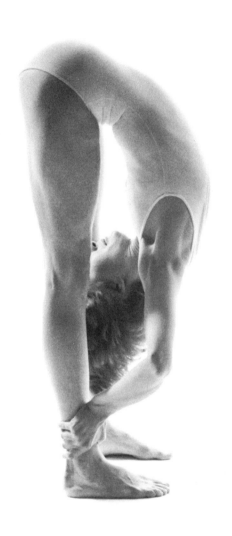

6 Then, as you exhale, contract your abdomen, bend your elbows, and bring your head toward your knees. Don't force your head down with your arms, but let the contraction pull you.

7 Relax as you inhale. Repeat Step 6.

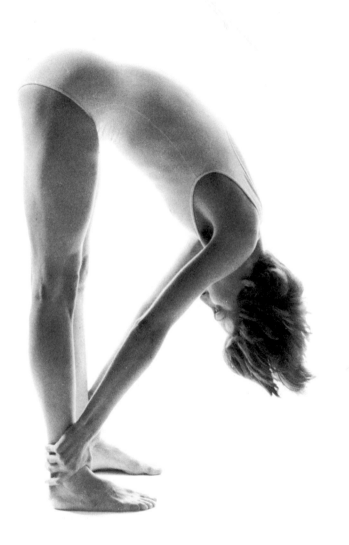

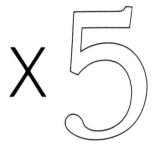

Do the exercise five times.

You may find it difficult at first to grasp your ankles or to bring your head to your knees, but with time your back and hamstrings should become more flexible. Don't force yourself in this exercise, but try to keep your shoulders relaxed. The only tension should be in your contraction, and you should feel a strong but not unpleasant pull up the backs of your legs and along the spine.

EXERCISE 30 PERFECT POSTURE

This is what it's all about: good posture, good looks, good spirits.

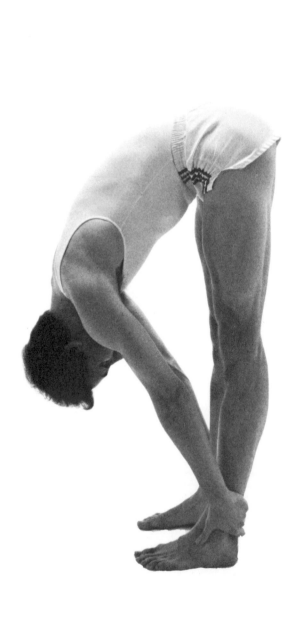

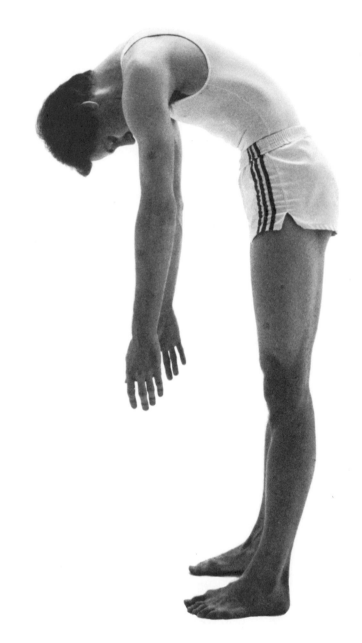

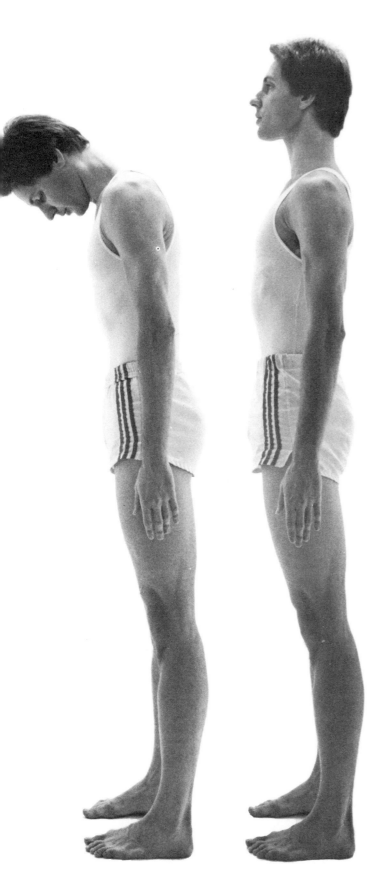

1 Starting from the last repetition of the previous exercise, inhale and release your ankles. Let your arms and hands hang.

2 Exhale and contract your abdomen. Now, using your pelvis like the reel on a fishing rod, slowly roll yourself up to a standing position, *one vertebra at a time.*

3 Keep bringing your weight forward and your pelvis under; let your arms and head hang relaxed until you're *all* the way up. Your tailbone should pull down as your spine rolls up.

4 Finally, let your head come up; stand straight and relaxed.

5 Now, breathe rhythmically, keeping your chest lifted, your shoulders down and relaxed. Place your weight lightly on the balls of your feet; don't lock your knees. Make your neck long — think about touching the ceiling with the top of your head. Inhale. Feel your knees in place directly over your feet, your hips in place directly over your knees, your spine long, your arms relaxed at your sides, your ears reaching upwards. On the exhale, contract the abdomen and slightly pull your pelvis under.

Inhale. . . .

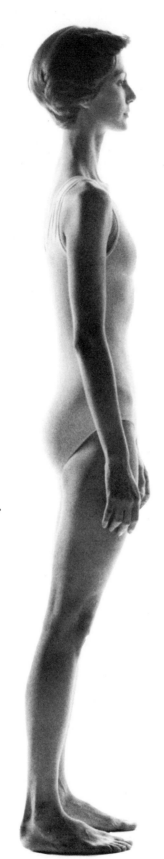

Exhale. . . .   There.

Natural Living

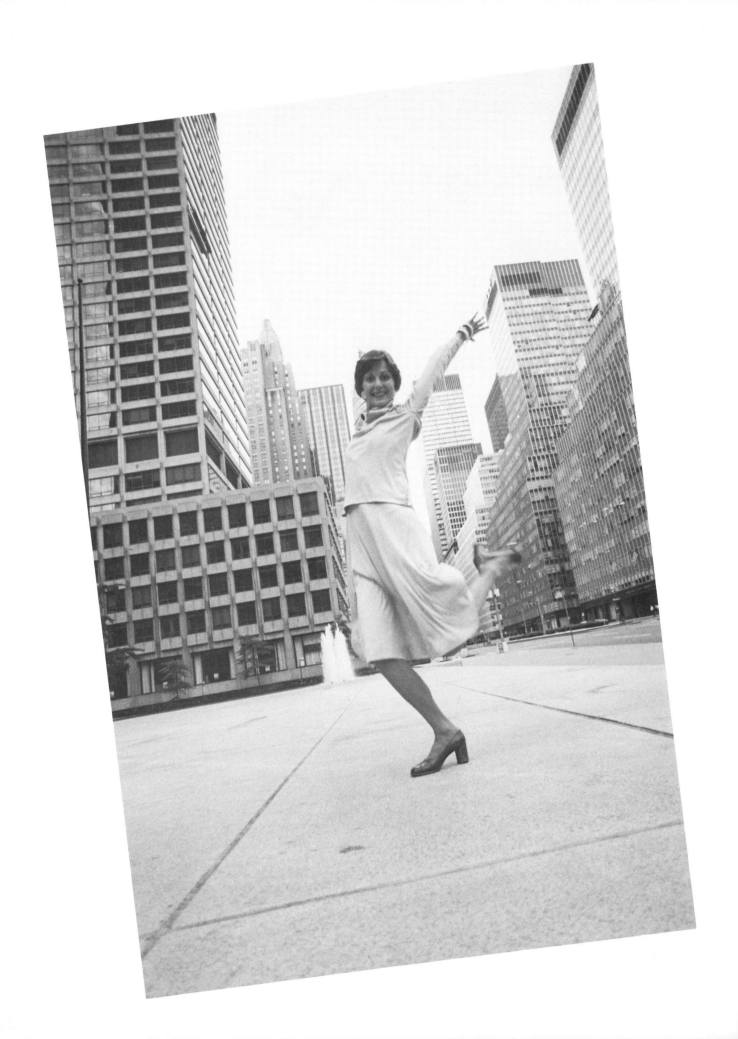

The Nickolaus Technique doesn't stop with EXERCISE 30, of course: The hour you spend on the exercises would be all but wasted if it weren't for the effect on the way you move and feel after you leave the exercise mat. Over a period of time, the Technique will naturally develop your musculature, strength, and flexibility, but at the same time it will deepen your understanding of how your body functions, and what it feels like when it is aligned correctly and moving as an organic unit. And the Technique teaches you how to nourish your body so that you look and feel at your peak.

In every waking moment, you can employ the principles of the Nickolaus Technique: the placement of the abdominal muscles, lower back, shoulders, and so on. When you move, you'll use your muscles efficiently and naturally. You may even find that you're eating more sensibly, since a good exercise program relieves stress you might otherwise relieve by overeating and puts you in touch with your body, so you instinctively watch your diet more carefully.

At first, you'll have to remind yourself of the way all that's supposed to feel, but with time your body will, in a sense, begin to exercise itself: Because you're walking, moving, breathing, and even eating correctly, everything you do will tend to reinforce the exercises. It will come to seem unnatural if you're not moving correctly.

How does it happen? When you complete a Nickolaus class or home workout, your body is aligned and in tune with itself. In the beginning, however, that feeling won't last long without conscious effort. As one of the instructors remarks, "You can walk out of a class totally up, and as you walk down the street, you can almost feel your shoulders sag and the muscle memory fade."

How, then, do you hold on to that memory?

For a start, try beginning each morning with a simplified, ten-minute warm-up that reminds your muscles what they've learned and puts you in gear for the day. It will help to flush out the carbon dioxide that accumulates in your lungs and body during sleep, replace it with fresh oxygen, and start your circulation going properly.

You can tailor your warm-up to your specific requirements—whether you're trying to limber up for sports or jogging or just trying to wake up in the morning—by selecting a combination of exercises that work on the areas you want to work on. Do them more quickly than you would if you were working on the complete sequence of the Nickolaus Technique, and always start with the first four exercises of the sequence. Like this:

1 Lie flat on your back and start with BREATHING (EXERCISE 1). Take at least five deep breaths; then bring one knee up to your chest and go directly into . . .

2 FOOT CIRCLES (EXERCISE 2). Do five in each direction, inhaling and exhaling more quickly than you would if you were trying to relax. Switch legs and repeat. Now go right on to . . .

3 FOOT FLEX (EXERCISE 3). Five inhale/exhales for each foot. Without pause . . .

4 SINGLE LEG STRETCH (EXERCISE 4). Do this fairly briskly, five times for each leg. Now you're limbered up and can go on to whatever combination of exercises seems right to prepare you for what you want to do. A good circulation-stimulator that will also stretch the back and hamstrings and Achilles tendon—important for sports like tennis or jogging—is . . .

5 DOUBLE LEG STRETCH (EXERCISE 5), done briskly five times. Since you're going more quickly in the warm-up than you would normally, make this slight variation to protect your back from strain: Extend your legs straight up toward the ceiling, rather than at an angle. Do this five times before straightening out your legs on the floor and doing a ROLL-UP to a sitting position with your arms over your head. Now . . .

6 Do the SITTING ARM AND LEG STRETCH (EXERCISE 6) five times, and after the fifth stretch . . .

7 Continue with the SITTING LOWER BACK STRETCH (EXERCISE 7), also done five times. Whatever combination of exercises you choose to warm up with, try finishing with . . .

8 SMALL BRIDGE (EXERCISE 8). One of the Nickolaus instructors calls this "a portable workout," because it contracts the stomach muscles, stretches the thighs, tightens the buttocks, and gently works the muscles of the lower back—all the things that the thirty exercises of the Nickolaus Technique have been developed to do. Five repetitions of this exercise at the close of your warm-up will tone and stimulate you, getting you ready for the day ahead.

This warm-up—or any other sequence that you might design for yourself—won't be easy, no matter how quick or simplified it is. Nor can a brief warm-up replace the complete sequence of the Nickolaus Technique. But it *is* a useful way of reminding your body of what it is learning from the Nickolaus Technique, and of keeping you from tightening up during the day.

You can also consciously check your body during the day: Are my shoulders tense when I sit at my desk? While I'm waiting for a bus, does the line of my body feel the way it does during PERFECT POSTURE? As I walk, am I breathing from the abdominal area, rather than high up in the chest?

Attention to breathing is especially important in daily life. As noted earlier, correct, relaxed, deep breathing can affect the way you react to stress, even the extent to which you're able to control your moods. In physical terms alone, the kind of breathing basic to the Nickolaus Technique is actually an effective lower abdominal exercise: The steady expansion and contraction will firm and strengthen the muscles of that area.

Similarly, holding the back in correct alignment will gradually strengthen the supporting muscles of the back; walking with a flexible, articulated foot will help the muscles of the leg and knee; keeping shoulders down, chest high, will develop the pectorals.

All that may sound as if moving through the day might become a pretty self-conscious progress. Remember, though, it's only at first that you have to remind yourself of what your body does — and only because most of us are so out of touch with our bodies. Eventually, the Nickolaus Technique will "teach" your body what easy, natural, flexible movement feels like.

It's especially important to apply the principles of the Nickolaus Technique to physical exertion that's out of the ordinary, from moving heavy furniture to dancing all night in a discotheque. For any activity you can imag-ine, correct body alignment and effective use of the abdominal muscles are essential.

Becoming aware of those crucial factors is a three-step process. First, as you do the exercises of the Nickolaus Technique, *think* about them. That may sound like obvious advice, but it's entirely possible to go through the movements of the Technique in an automatic, "technical" manner, without really considering what your body is doing. Or you may become so preoccupied with executing the movement correctly that you forget what its purpose is.

It takes practice, but keep trying to make a connection in your mind between what goes on subjectively — your feelings about what's happening with your body — during an exercise, and the objective movements you are executing. This is the first step in transferring the principles of the Nickolaus Technique into your daily life.

The second step is to expand the process and, as you walk, reach, run, bend, stand, and sit, try to discover in what way those movements do and do not resemble what you feel while you're on the exercise mat doing the Nickolaus Technique.

Finally, put it all together so that gradually your day-to-day movements come to feel more and more like the movements of the Nickolaus Technique.

Sound rather theoretical? It would be, if it were just a matter of thinking about it. But we're talking about something you *do*. For example, deep breathing alone can be a powerful reinforcement of the Nickolaus Technique. Say you're at work, sitting at your desk; around the middle of the afternoon you realize you feel tired, tense, and physically dragged out. Take a couple of minutes to concentrate on your breathing, consciously bringing your abdominal muscles into play, and filling your lungs from the bottom up, as in EXERCISE 1 (and, indeed, throughout the

Nickolaus Technique). See if you don't sit straighter, feel more relaxed, and have more energy.

If you can do them without creating a scene in the office, the HEAD ROLLS (EXERCISE 14) can be combined with abdominal breathing, as they are during the Technique. This exercise relaxes and stretches the areas where tension is most likely to accumulate as a result of sedentary work like typing.

Suppose you're standing around waiting for a bus, a subway, or a date. How close are you to PERFECT POSTURE? Is your chest lifted; are your shoulders down? As you exhale, do you contract your abdomen and slightly pull your pelvis under?

Or it's moving day, and you're hauling furniture around. As you lift a heavy object, do you inhale in preparation for the exertion and release your breath evenly as you lift? Or do you tense up, locking the breath inside? Depending on the answer, it's possible to go through a day of fairly strenuous physical effort and feel either invigorated or exhausted at the end of it.

It is through this attention to your body in specific moments of physical activity and inactivity that you can begin to grasp the principles of the Nickolaus Technique in relation to daily life.

Above all, those principles can assist you as you prepare for any kind of athletic activity: jogging, tennis, skiing, handball, golf, badminton, or even a brisk walk. At the very least, before going onto a tennis court or jogging track, it would be smart to prepare by taking a few minutes to do the BREATHING. Even better would be the BREATHING followed by a sequence of exercises involving stretching and extension — say, 1 through 8. Specific exercises can be used to work on special problems that crop up in connection with sports or recreational activities. The LEG LIFTS, for instance, are good for knee problems. Where the problems are serious, you should of course seek your physician's advice about which exercises might be helpful.

As you start paying more attention to the way you look and feel, you may discover you are thinking more about your diet. It's natural. Not only do you want to look your best — and for some people this means losing weight as well as firming muscles — but you want to feel your best, and you can't feel your best if you're not getting a nourishing, efficient diet. How can you build this into your daily routine?

The exercises in the Nickolaus Technique improve coordination, make you feel better, and improve your looks, grace, and ease of movement. They will not, in and of themselves, take pounds off your frame. They can help you keep your stomach flat and your legs and arms firm, while each movement of the Technique will burn up at least a few of your extra calories — but for people with weight problems this is not enough. A vigorous routine of daily exercise may be of great help; but it must be combined with proper eating habits to take weight off and keep it off.

For a start, throw away the salt shaker and sugar bowl, give up soft drinks, avoid fatty meats of all kinds, and eat more vegetables, fruit, skimmed milk, and fish.

Avoid fried foods, including fish and potatoes — though both are fine if boiled or broiled.

From hard experience, most weight-watchers learn that a person should not only cut down on sugar, but aim to eliminate it altogether by tapering off gradually, then switching to sugar substitutes or honey. Cakes and pastries or candies made with sugar are for special occasions only.

Better yet, develop the habit of substituting fresh fruit or vegetable snacks for coffee breaks and desserts. Raw fruits and vegetables are important because they add necessary vitamins, minerals, and bulk to your diet. If possible, though, you should pass up snacks in favor of three attractively prepared meals a day — and you should be careful not to miss one. One of the worst things that someone watching weight can do is to skip a meal. When this occurs, the tendency is for the hunger to build, and for the dieter to become increasingly aware that a meal was missed and to compensate by eating even more.

The key, then, is a well-served meal prepared with imagination — a meal in which you have three or four different items on your plate, including one or two vegetables, a small portion of fish or lean meat (veal or chicken are best), and a large salad with a minimum of dressing. Include as great a variety of food as possible, within reasonable bounds, so there is enough bulk to make you feel satisfied at the conclusion of the meal, though the meal itself may not be more than 1200 calories.

Essentially, if you are determined to improve your eating habits, the only way to go about it so that you can keep it up on a daily basis is to decide you must change your lifestyle when it comes to food — and then stick to the change. Go over this simple checklist of essential vitamins and minerals. Are you getting enough of them in your diet? Do you know what foods they're found in? And do you know what they do for you?

VITAMIN A Found in apricots, liver, eggs, butter, whole milk, deep-yellow vegetables like carrots, deep-green leafy vegetables; it helps in the development of skin and teeth and eyes.

VITAMIN D Found in sunshine, egg yolks, vitamin-D milk, butter, fortified margarine, liver, tuna, salmon, fish-liver oils; it promotes the absorption of calcium in your body for strong bones and teeth.

VITAMIN E Found in fresh whole-grain wheat products, vegetable oils, liver, beans and peas, butter, eggs, leafy green vegetables; it prevents the deterioration of fats and oils in stored foods, and may also play a role in improving circulation (although there is no definitive information on this point as yet).

VITAMIN C Found in citrus fruits, green and yellow peppers, other fresh vegetables, and liver; it aids in the normal development of body tissues such as bone, teeth, and blood vessels, and of collagen (a protein that supports body structures like bone and tendon and helps give skin its elasticity).

VITAMIN B$_1$ (Thiamine) Found in whole grains, liver, heart, kidney, fish and meats (especially pork), nuts, legumes such as peas, beans, and lentils, milk; it helps your body use its carbohydrates, aids in the energy-releasing chemical reactions in the body.

FOLIC ACID Found in liver, leafy vegetables, whole grains, nuts, legumes; it is an important component in the formation of chemicals for the nuclei of all body cells and thus aids in promoting cell replacement in skin, mucous membranes, and blood.

VITAMIN B$_2$ (Riboflavin) Found in milk, cheese, liver, kidneys, eggs, nuts, legumes, leafy vegetables, lean meat, whole grains; it helps your body use its oxygen properly.

VITAMIN B$_3$ (Niacin) Found in whole-grain cereals and breads, eggs, meat, liver, nuts, legumes; it assists the chemical helpers needed for many essential energy-yielding reactions and for proper nervous-system function.

VITAMIN B$_6$ Found in liver, meats, leafy green vegetables, whole grains, bananas; it aids in normal red blood cell formation and helps the body metabolize its amino acids (the building blocks of protein) and fats.

VITAMIN B$_{12}$ Found in liver, kidneys, meat, fish, eggs, shellfish, milk products; it is important for the synthesizing of nucleic acids (the chemicals that form the nuclei of your body cells) and for the building of red blood cells, and it aids in the function of the nervous system.

PANTOTHENIC ACID Found in yeast, liver, eggs, whole grains, nuts, legumes; it is a key component in the metabolism of protein, carbohydrates, and fats, as well as in the formation of important hormones and nerve-regulating substances.

You should also be getting enough Vitamin K (for your eyes), calcium (for strong bones and teeth), phosphorus, iron (for red blood cells), magnesium, iodine, sodium, potassium, zinc, and other minerals. Check with your doctor for a list of the federally established Minimum Daily Requirements for vitamins and minerals, and make sure you get them. If you eat properly, not only will you look better, you'll feel better — and feeling good is what the Nickolaus Technique is all about.

If you merely do the thirty exercises for an hour, twice a week, the Nickolaus Technique will eventually make itself felt throughout your daily life. But with conscious, sustained effort, you can hasten and intensify the process. More is involved than simply understanding that your body used to move one way and now it's moving differently. What you're approaching is an understanding of how your body affects the total quality of your daily life.

Consider this. We spend years training our minds in school, high school, college. Yet for most of us there is no equivalent training for the body. A strange disporportion, since in a literal sense it is our bodies that carry our minds — or at least, our heads — through life.

Equally strange is the attitude that many of us learn toward our bodies as a result of this unbalanced emphasis. Qualities of the mind are prized in our society; but, except in the most superficial way, we tend to look down on the body: It fails us, it gets sick, it grows old. We admire the physically fit body, we may applaud it in performance, whether artistic or athletic, but we do not truly respect it. It's not difficult to find many examples of people who dislike and resent their own bodies and reveal that attitude by ignoring them, feeding them indifferently, giving them insufficient rest, or silencing them with drugs.

The Nickolaus Technique addresses itself squarely to those twin problems: lack of education about the body, and lack of identification with it. Through applying what is described in this book to your life, you will not only increase your stamina, range of motion, and general physical well-being. You will — again, literally speaking — "change your mind."

A Nickolaus student summed it up well: "People think exercise is a cosmetic thing, that it will make their bodies look better. Well it does, but I've also found a great deal of my life has improved as a result of the Nickolaus Technique. Once the exercises start making you feel better and look better, you start feeling different about yourself. In a real way, your whole life feels better."